Andréia Guerra Siman
M. de Oliveira Fani Amaro

Nursing Management in the Context of Quality

Andréia Guerra Siman
M. de Oliveira Fani Amaro

Nursing Management in the Context of Quality

The nurse's managerial work: from Primary Health Care to the Hospital environment

ScienciaScripts

Imprint

Any brand names and product names mentioned in this book are subject to trademark, brand or patent protection and are trademarks or registered trademarks of their respective holders. The use of brand names, product names, common names, trade names, product descriptions etc. even without a particular marking in this work is in no way to be construed to mean that such names may be regarded as unrestricted in respect of trademark and brand protection legislation and could thus be used by anyone.

Cover image: www.ingimage.com

This book is a translation from the original published under ISBN 978-613-9-72879-4.

Publisher:
Sciencia Scripts
is a trademark of
Dodo Books Indian Ocean Ltd. and OmniScriptum S.R.L publishing group

120 High Road, East Finchley, London, N2 9ED, United Kingdom
Str. Armeneasca 28/1, office 1, Chisinau MD-2012, Republic of Moldova, Europe
Printed at: see last page
ISBN: 978-620-6-19588-7

PART I

Presentation

This work is a collection of articles organized with several authors.

CHAPTER 1

THE PROGRAM TO IMPROVE ACCESS AND QUALITY IN PRIMARY CARE FROM THE PERSPECTIVE OF NURSES: PERCEPTIONS AND COMPLICATING ASPECTS

Marilane de Oliveira Fani Amaro

Camilo Amaro de Carvalho
Greicy Kelly Franco Tavares
Thaís dos Santos Pinheiro

INTRODUCTION

The healthcare model in Brazil has been undergoing restructuring since the creation of the Unified Health System (SUS) in the late 1980s. To this end, it has Primary Health Care (PHC) as its main guiding element, currently based on the Family Health Strategy (FHS). This, in turn, aims to organize the Health Care Networks serving all citizens holistically and with quality[1] .

Users require care to be provided by a multi-professional team, characterised by the presence of professionals from different areas of training and levels of education. It is important to ensure that the care is provided to the clientele in accordance with the principles of the SUS[2] .

Among the multiprofessional team, the nurse is included, responsible for providing comprehensive care to users, acting in the management and coordination of the actions of community health workers (CHWs). In addition, he promotes continuing education and participates in the management of inputs necessary for the health unit to function properly offering quality care to the community[3] .

In the context of the quality of care in PHC, it is important to implement means to evaluate the services offered in PHC. In 2011, the Ministry of Health (MS) created through Ordinance No. 1.654 GM/MS, the Primary Care Access and Quality Improvement Program (PMAQ-AB) aimed at institutionalizing the evaluation of Primary Care, aiming to induce the expansion of access and improvement of quality[4] .

The PMAQ-AB is divided into four phases. The first phase is the adherence to the program through the contractualization of commitments and indicators. It should be voluntary, as it is based on the assumption that the motivation and proactivity of the participants are key factors for success. The second stage deals with the development of the set of actions that should

be carried out by the teams, subdivided into four sub-phases: self-evaluation, monitoring, continuing education and institutional support. The third consists of the external evaluation in which the conditions of access and quality are explored and, finally, the fourth phase is characterized by the recontractualization, consisting of a process of pact between the teams and the municipality with the development of new standards and quality indicators[5] .

When it comes to health management, continuous assessment facilitates decision making by making it more coherent since it is possible to point out in detail the problems detected and reorganize the work process. This leads to the achievement of the proposed goals and improves care for the community. Therefore, the nurse as a member of the minimum team in the PCU with the aforementioned attributions has the ability to perform actions for the benefit of users and in an integrated manner with the entire team[6] .

Considering the relevance of nurses as members of the PHC team, professionals who have a work process that directly influences the quality of care, the guiding question of this research was: how was the implementation of the PMAQ-AB from the nurses' perspective? Thus, this study aims to understand the implementation of the PMAQ-AB from the perspective of PHC nurses, regarding the team's adherence, the difficulties for implementation and the benefits resulting from the program.

METHODS

This is a descriptive research with a qualitative approach. The definition for the qualitative research line occurred due to its characteristic of working with values, beliefs, representations, habits, attitudes and opinions, and for being an interpretative-formative type of investigation, which seeks the understanding of the researched theme, favouring the discovery process, by means of analysis, synthesis of ideas and concepts, with involvement of emotional and contextual aspects[7] .

The study scenario was a municipality in Zona da Mata Mineira that has 17 family health teams, providing coverage of approximately 65% of the population. The undergraduate nursing students of a public university are inserted in this scenario, developing practical activities and curricular internships, with care and management actions of disease prevention and health promotion, which contributed to the choice of the scenario.

Inclusion criteria were: to work as a nurse in the municipality's FHS, regardless of how long they have been working there. The exclusion criteria were nurses away from the job for any reason. During data collection, one professional was on holiday, one was on leave and three refused to participate. Therefore, the research participants were: 12 nurses.

Data were collected in the period from April to August 2016, through interviews with a semi-structured script. The interviews were recorded and later transcribed in full. The guiding questions discussed the form of adherence of the team to the program, the difficulties for implementation and the benefits arising from the PMAQ-AB for the nurse coordinator of the unit.

The interviews were recorded in the workplace, according to the availability of the nurses, in a reserved room so that participants could expose their experiences calmly and safely. These lasted an average of 30 minutes. All interviews were recorded and transcribed in full. To preserve anonymity, the nurses are represented by the letters ENF preceded by the number corresponding to the order in which the interviews were conducted, namely: ENF1, ENF2, ENF3, and so on.

For data analysis it was performed the content analysis technique[8] , which proposes a sequence for analysis based on the following steps: pre analysis, material exploration and treatment of results, inference and interpretation. Thus, initially a floating and exhaustive reading of the material was carried out in order to have a familiarization with the text and obtain an understanding of what the subject sought to convey. Then we proceeded to the thematic selection, which consisted in identifying the nuclei of meaning, or semantically similar elements, for further categorization and analysis in the light of the literature. From the analysis, they could be grouped into three thematic categories: The process of adherence to the PMAQ-AB: perceptions of nurses; The PMAQ- AB as a tool in work planning and organization; Experiencing the PMAQ-AB: hindering aspects.

The study was conducted according to the standards of Resolution 466/2012 of the National Health Council, having been approved by the Ethics Committee on Research with Human Beings of the Federal University of Viçosa under CAAE n°: 43931315.0.0000.5153.

RESULTS AND DISCUSSION

After data collection, the profile of the research subjects was drawn, being 11 (91.7%) female. The professionals' age ranged between 28 and 52 years. Regarding the time of work in the institution the average was 9 years, with variation between 3 months and 6 years and as for the time of formation the average obtained was 9.6 years varying between 3 and 27 years and all had specialization in public health or collective health. The workload of all interviewees was 40 hours per week and none of the interviewees had other employment relationship.

The process of adherence to the PMAQ-AB: nurses' perceptions

Through the statements, it was found that the participants had difficulties in explaining how the process of implementation of the programme took place, explaining that such a fact occurred in a vertical way:

"What is this registration that you are talking about? Because I am a primary care nurse who is a PMAQ-AB member, so every team is enrolled. The secretariat enrolls all the units." (ENF02)

"In fact, we are not the ones who signed up. When they come to evaluate the municipality, then the system opens for the municipality to register the units that are going to be evaluated. Then the health secretariat registers the professionals who are going to be evaluated." (ENF06)

"I am enrolled because I was forced. Even the unit that didn't want to register, the PMAQ had it there. So I was forced to register. But everyone here is registered." (ENF05)

Enrollment in PMAQ-AB is formalized through the Department of Health and Human Services' Program Management System (Sistema de Gestão de Programas do Departamento de AB), which takes place in three stages: expression of interest by the municipal manager, adherence and contractualization of the health care teams, and adherence and contractualization by the municipal manager[5].

Prior to the beginning of the program, it is necessary to clarify what the PMAQ-AB consists of and what its objectives are, thus allowing the opening of a space that promotes dialogue, problematization of reality and subsequent contractualization of the teams. Most participants in this study stated that the implementation occurred in a vertical manner, diverging from the voluntary character recommended by the MS.

Other studies converge to the same finding. In the Federal District, the absence of choice for adherence to the program was highlighted[9] and another research conducted in Ceará highlighted that the process also occurred in a vertical manner without any clarification and with precarious discussion about the PMAQ-AB, in addition, some teams that did not adhere for political issues due to partisan rivalry before the municipal manager[10].

It is suggested that the financial incentive received by the municipality after approval of adherence significantly influences the managers' decision to join the PMAQ-AB. Every month, 20% of the full value of the Quality Component of the Variable Primary Care Payment (Variable PAB) is transferred to each registered team .[5]

Moreover, the performance of the teams that are compulsorily enrolled in the program is questionable, since the motivation and proactivity of the professionals involved influence the outcome of health care, since it is necessary that there is protagonism of all involved. Voluntary adherence is associated with the idea that it will only be possible to intervene in the quality of services provided if health professionals and managers feel motivated to do so[11].

The PMAQ-AB as a tool for work planning and organization

The PMAQ-AB as a strategy to promote quality in health, allows the organization of services and sets standards aimed at continuous improvement of the PC, interfering directly in the work process of health teams. The participants' statements pointed out that the program helps in planning and organizing the work:

"...I realised people were more concerned about organisations. I think so it improved in terms of service provision, attention in some situations." (ENF05)

"Ah...I believe that users are better welcomed when we are more oriented, more organized with all service planning, I think it works better. "(ENF08)

"We are able to work more within the protocol, many situations that we did not do that primary care recommends, with the arrival of PMAQ we began to implement, to develop. "(ENF02)

"So the benefits of the programme is that poorly or well, I don't know what personal motivation each team member has, but poorly or well the improvement activities are executed." (ENF01)

The second phase of the PMAQ-AB (with emphasis on self-evaluation) and the third phase (external evaluation) of the program stand out as fundamental steps to identify the negative and positive points arising from the team itself and then the collection of information for analysis of both the work of health professionals and municipal managers.

The self-evaluation is considered as the part that will start the development phase. In it, the weaknesses and potentialities of the service are recognized by the team itself. The word "evaluation" is usually associated with punishments and negative aspects, but it should not be perceived in this way by professionals. It is a fundamental component so that one can problematize a certain situation and from there seek solutions. According to the statement made by the MH: *"[...] so that it can constitute a critical-reflective action, it is important that the self-evaluation is performed among peers, collectively, considering all the actors involved with primary care in its different spheres. Based on the result of the self-evaluation, situations that need to be reviewed and/or modified will be identified*[5] *"*.

The external evaluation performs a set of actions to examine the conditions of access and quality of all municipalities enrolled in the program. The PMAQ- AB certification process should be understood as a moment of recognition of the efforts of the teams and the municipal manager. From this, health teams can be classified into four categories: (I) unsatisfactory performance; (II) regular performance; (III) good performance; (IV) optimal performance. According to the classifications, over time it will be possible for the team itself to evaluate its performance during the program[5] .

A study analyzed the facilitating and limiting elements of external evaluation. It was pointed out as a positive point that the activities proposed by PMAQ-AB enhance the internal coordination of SUS and place the assessment and planning as elements that involve the team and management to the detriment of improving the quality and access to AB[12] . This finding addresses a common point with the present study since the participants report in their statements words such as "implant", "develop", "organized", "planning", "improvements" evidencing the changes made in PHC.

Cruz et al[13] points out that recognizing the inherent connections present between planning and evaluation, in addition to the relevance of these as guiding the work process, it is understood that there is an approximation of this practice to the idea of dynamization and consequent breaking of fragmented and bureaucratized planning and evaluation.

Therefore, the establishment of evaluation in the PCU has given way to a critical-reflexive practice of the actions taken by health teams, thus facilitating the development of action plans in order to improve what was previously detected as a failure.

Experiencing the PMAQ-AB: difficult aspects

This category shows the nurses' concern about the working conditions, which are presented as aspects that hinder the achievement of the goals proposed by the PMAQ-AB. They cited: the lack of material resources, the precariousness of the physical network, the inadequate quantity and high turnover of professionals. Such concerns are observed in the following statements:

"The great difficulty in implementing PMAQ is not charging, the great difficulty is the working conditions...it's coming here and sometimes I have to make a bandage and I don't have a bandage...then I have to go there and ask the user to buy it, because I only have gauze and adhesive tape, I also don't have ointment..." (ENF02)

"The working conditions, there is no way, there are no materials, there are not enough medicines to serve everyone, so I think it is a great difficulty. I even have micro areas that are uncovered". (ENF07)

"Suddenly I am well evaluated, but because of the physical structure, I don't know, sometimes there is mold there, then my unit already falls". (ENF07)

"The difficulties are infrastructure, lack of material, but that's it. Professional too, I have few professionals, so I don't provide 100% coverage and they directly change the doctor". (ENF12)

Despite the advances of the FHS in Brazil, many challenges affecting the quality of care still need to be overcome. According to the MS, through Ordinance No. 703 of 21 October 2011, the minimum number of professionals for a FHS team should be: one nurse, one nursing assistant and one doctor, responsible for a coverage area of up to 4,000 people. It is imperative that the number of CHAs cover 100% of the registered population, with a maximum of 750 people for each in a total of 12 professionals per team[14]

Moreover, according to Mayer et al[15] it has been observed in different studies that the high turnover of professionals in the PCU is present and can be related to objective and subjective aspects. They mention the precarious contractual relationship, the political relationship between professional and manager, and professional fulfillment. Such aspects reflect directly on users, since there is no establishment of bonds, a key element when it comes to PHC.

In addition, the ambience and availability of materials needed to perform various procedures compromise the access and quality of care. A place suitable to receive all users with comfort and privacy, allowing greater interaction with the team, influences the care and satisfaction of both those who offer services and those who receive them. Garcia et al[16] cites: *"When adapting the concept of ambience to the health area, it highlights the great importance for the configuration of the service in its concrete structural aspect, as well as in the interaction and bonds with service users and their families, and as a facilitating tool of the work process, in which it should ensure the right to privacy and respect for individuality, enabling the production of subjectivities, translating into a space that instigates the reflection of practices and ways of operating in it, contributing to the transformation of existing paradigms."*

In a survey conducted in Paraná to evaluate the satisfaction and dissatisfaction of PHC workers, the deficit of work tools and PHCU structures was elected, emphasizing the precariousness of the physical area as the most significant condition interfering with the work process[17].

Donabedian et al[18] mentions that the structure contributes to the development of care processes, reflecting on their results and playing a central role in improving the quality of services. This is directly related to what is called the "stable conditions of health services", meaning the material and human resources, the physical context, the organizational model and the instruments that involve health actions.

In short, it is clear the importance that the ambience and the structuring of the team have in the context of PHC and how these factors interfere in the work process and in the way that health services are offered to users impacting directly on health quality.

CONCLUSIONS

The study concluded that the process of adherence and contractualization to the program for improving access and quality in Primary Care occurred in a vertical manner. It is believed that political strategies are one of the main reasons for this, since the federal government sends financial subsidies from the moment of its approval.

The aspect of verticalization may be detrimental in the implementation of consecutive phases of the program, since its hiring should be voluntary, so that then, it could create a space for dialogue about the goals that will be implemented in view, clearly, all the objectives of the PMAQ-AB.

Moreover, barriers to the improvement of health services were cited, such as the physical structure of the units, the amount of human resources less than recommended and the high turnover of health professionals. These factors are related to the professional's dissatisfaction, compromising the performance of their activities.

It is believed that although the phase of adherence and contractualization has occurred in a compulsory way and because it is a relatively new government strategy, with challenges to be faced, the interviewees recognize the positive effects of PMAQ-AB in their daily practices. However, the lack of further studies on the subject hinders further discussions.

REFERENCES

1. Feitosa RMM, Paulino AA, Júnior JOSL, Oliveira KKD de, Freitas RJM de, Silva WF da. Changes offered by the National Program for Improving Access and Quality of Primary Care.

Saúde Soc 2016;25(3):821-829.

2. Silva MVS da, Miranda GBN, Andrade MA de. Sentidos atribuídos à integralidade: entre o que é preconizado e vivido na equipe multidisciplinar. Interface (Botucatu) 2017;21(62): 589599.

3. Brazil. Ministério da Saúde. Secretariat of Health Care. Department of Basic Care. Política Nacional de Atenção Básica. Brasília; 2006.

4. Brazil. Ordinance No. 1654 of 19 July 2011. Institui, no âmbito do Sistema Único de Saúde, o Programa Nacional de Melhoria do Acesso e da Qualidade da Atenção Básica (PMAQ-AB) e o Incentivo Financeiro do PMAQ-AB, denominado Componente de Qualidade do Piso de Atenção Básica Variável - PAB Variável. Diário Oficial da União 2011; 19 Jul.

5. Brazil. Ministério da Saúde; Secretária de Atenção à saúde, Departamento de Atenção Básica. Programa Nacional de Melhoria do Acesso e da Qualidade da Atenção Básica (PMAQ): manual instructivo. 1ª ed. Brasília; 2012.

6. Jesus AS de, Cardoso TSG, Vilela ABA, Nery AA. O enfermeiro no contexto do programa nacional de melhoria do acesso e de qualidade da atenção básica (PMAQ): relato de experiência Rev. Saúde. Com 2015;11(2):193-200.

7. Minayo MCS. The challenge of knowledge: qualitative health research. 12a Edição. São Paulo, Rio de Janeiro: Hucitec, Abrasco; 2010.

8. Bardin L. Content Analysis. São Paulo: Edições 70, 2011.

9. Lopes EAA, Scherer MDA, Costa AM. O Programa Nacional de Melhoria do Acesso e da Qualidade da Atenção Básica e a organização dos processos de trabalho. Tempus, actas de saúde colet, 2015;9(2):237-250.

10. Linhares PH A, Lira GV, Albuquerque IMN. Avaliação do Programa Nacional de Melhoria do Acesso e da Qualidade da Atenção Básica no estado do Ceará. Saúde debate 2014; 38(spe):195-208.

11. Ministério da Saúde (BR). Programa Nacional de Melhoria do Acesso e da Qualidade da Atenção Básica (PMAQ). Manual Instrutivo 3° Ciclo. Brasília: Ministry of Health;2015-2016.

12. Melo DC, Rocha AARM, Aleluia IRS. External evaluation of PMAQ-AB: facilitating and limiting elements in a capital city of the Brazilian Northeast. Rev. Gestão & Saúde 2017;08(1):3-17.

13. Cruz MM da, Souza RBC de, Torres RMC, Abreu DMFA, Reis AC, Gonçalves AL. Uses of planning and self-assessment in the work processes of Family Health teams in Primary Care. Saúde Debate 2014;38(spe):124-139.

14. Brazil. Ordinance No. 703 of 21 October 2011. Estabelece normas para o cadastramento, no

Sistema de Cadastro Nacional de Estabelecimentos de Saúde (SCNES), das novas equipes que serão part da Estratégia de Saúde da Família (ESF). Diário Oficial da União 2011; 21 Oct.

15. Mayer BLD, Huppes RE, Silva FS da, Weiller TH, Poll MA. Primary care health professionals and the evaluation: integrative literature review. Saúde (Santa Maria) 2015;41(1):19-28.

16. Garcia ANP, Andrade MAC, Contarato PC, Tristão FI,Rocha EMS, Rabello AE, Lima RCD. Ambiência na Estratégia Saúde da Família. Vigil. sanit. debate 2015;3(2):36-41.

17. Lima L de, Pires DElP de, Forte ECN, Medeiros F. Satisfação e insatisfação no trabalho de profissionais de saúde da atenção básica. Esc. Anna Nery 2014; 18(1):17-24.

18. Donabedian A, Wheeler HRC, Wysze-Wianski L. Quality, Cost, and Health: An Integrative Model. Med. Care 20(10): 1975-92, 1982.

CHAPTER 2

QUALITY IN PRIMARY CARE: PERCEPTIONS OF COMMUNITY HEALTH WORKERS ON PMAQ-AB

Marilane de Oliveira Fani Amaro
Camilo Amaro de Carvalho Rita
de Cássia Vaz Barral Thaís dos
Santos Pinheiro

INTRODUCTION

Since the creation of the Unified Health System (SUS) in the late 1980s, Brazil has been undergoing a restructuring of its healthcare system, with Primary Health Care (PHC) as its main guiding element, currently based on the Family Health Strategy (FHS). Thus, it aims at health promotion and protection, prevention of diseases, diagnosis, treatment, rehabilitation and harm reduction, responding to the needs of the population in order to develop holistic care .[1]

For this, it is necessary to incorporate a collective, inter and multiprofessional approach to actions, requiring from the professionals skills and abilities for the development of tasks that include both the care to the individual, family and community, as well as the activities of planning and management of the service[2] .

Among the multiprofessional team, since the institution of the Community Health Agent Program (PACS), the presence of the Community Health Agent (CHA) is necessary, selected in the community to act together with the population, thus providing subsidies for the construction of a new model of health care, since its function is to integrate users to health services, uniting technical and popular knowledge and thus impacting on the reorganization and quality of the same[3,4] .

The professional attribution of the CHA is translated into disease prevention and health promotion, which can be through home or community actions, of individual or collective nature, and which are developed in accordance with the SUS guidelines in the context of Primary Health Care (BHC)[3] .

Due to the changes that have occurred in recent decades, the Ministry of Health (MH) created in 2011, through Ordinance No. 1.654 GM/MS, the Primary Care Access and Quality Improvement Program (PMAQ-AB) aiming to institutionalize the evaluation of Primary Care. The aim is thus to induce the expansion of access and improvement of quality, allowing greater transparency and effectiveness of actions, associating the three spheres of SUS management (MS, state and municipal managers) .[5]

The PMAQ-AB is divided into four phases, the first of which is the adherence phase, through the contractualization of commitments and indicators. The second stage is the development of the set of actions that will be undertaken by the teams and is organized into four dimensions (self-evaluation, monitoring, continuing education and institutional support). The third stage consists of the external evaluation, where a set of actions will be carried out to assess the conditions of access and quality in all the municipalities. The fourth phase is the re-contractualization that consists of a unique pacting process of the teams and municipalities with the increase of new standards and quality indicators[6].

To obtain better results and the consequent affirmation of the effectiveness of the PCU as the gateway to health services, it is necessary that the agreed indicators are achieved according to the established goals. The competitiveness generated from this, increases the pressure suffered by CHWs to meet the goals, culminating with wear and tear and psychological suffering, directly influencing the quality of care[7].

In addition, the CHWs are inserted in an environment where there is no clarity in the delimitation of their practices, competencies and skills, interfering in the way this professional acts and possibly impacting health care. Thus, it is assumed that the PMAQ-AB is not widely known by CHWs, resulting in a misconception of the program.

Given the relevance of CHWs as part of the work process in PHC directly influencing the quality of care provided as well as the objectives of PMAQ-AB, the guiding question of this research was: what is the perception of CHWs regarding the implementation of PMAQ-AB? Thus, this study aims to assess the CHWs' perception of the PMAQ-BA in a municipality of Minas Gerais, Brazil.

METHODS

This is a descriptive research with a qualitative approach. The definition for the qualitative research line occurred due to its characteristic of working with values, beliefs, representations, habits, attitudes and opinions, and for being an interpretative-formative type of investigation, which seeks the understanding of the researched theme, favouring the discovery process, by means of analysis, synthesis of ideas and concepts, with involvement of emotional and contextual aspects[8].

The study scenario was in a municipality in Zona da Mata Mineira. It has 17 family health teams, providing coverage of approximately 65% of the population. In this health context, the undergraduate nursing students of a university are inserted, developing practical activities and curricular internships with care and management actions for disease prevention and health promotion.

The inclusion criteria were: to act as CHWs in the ESF of the municipality in question, regardless of how long they have been working in the position. The exclusion criterion was ACS away from the job for any reason. During data collection, seven professionals were on holiday and 27 refused to participate. Therefore, the research participants were 47 CHWs.

Data were collected in the period from April to August 2016, through semi-structured interviews. The interviews were recorded and later transcribed in full. The guiding questions discussed the understanding about the PMAQ-AB, benefits and difficulties in its implementation and what is the role of the CHW as a member of the health team in the PMAQ-AB.

The interviews were recorded at their workplace, according to the availability of the CHWs, in a reserved room so that participants could expose their experiences calmly and safely. To preserve anonymity, the CHWs were represented by the letters ACS preceded by the number corresponding to the order in which the interviews were conducted, namely: ACS1, ACS2, ACS3, and so on.

For qualitative analysis of the results it was performed the content analysis technique[9] , which proposes a sequence for analysis based on the following steps: pre-analysis, material exploration and treatment of results, inference and interpretation. Thus, initially a floating and exhaustive reading of the interview questions was carried out in order to become familiar with the text and obtain an understanding of what the subject sought to convey. Then we proceeded to the thematic selection, which consisted in identifying the nuclei of meaning, or semantically similar elements, for further categorization. Finally, they were analysed in the light of the literature.

The study was conducted according to the norms of Resolution 466/2012 of the National Health Council, having been approved by the Ethics Committee for Research with Human Beings of the Federal University of Viçosa under CAAE n°:4393115.0.0000.5153.

RESULTS AND DISCUSSION

After data collection, the profile of the research participants was drawn, with 46 (97.9%) being female. The professionals' age ranged between 25 and 51 years, with an average of 36.29 years. Regarding the time of work in the institution, the average was 5.8 years, varying between eight months and ten years. As for the workload, all interviewees worked 40 hours per week and none of them had any other employment relationship.

After analysis of the interviews, the following categories emerged: Expressions and impressions about PMAQ-AB from the perspective of CHWs; PMAQ-AB: Limitations experienced by CHWs and Potentialities of PMAQ-AB from the perspective of CHWs.

Expressions and impressions of the PMAQ-AB from the perspective of CHWs

The statements below demonstrate the CHAs' perception of the programme:

"That it is a government programme to give more quality in the service, access for patients in the PSF." (ACS9)

"To my knowledge it is a programme for improving the quality of health care." (ACS16)

"It's a programme to improve access and quality." (ACS14)

It is noticed that the CHAs' understanding is limited to the definition of the concept of the program as a strategy for evaluation of the PCU aimed at improving quality and access. Therefore, reflecting on *quality in health* assumes extreme relevance. At first, it is about how the services have been perceived by users. In order to assess quality, the context in which the service is inserted should be considered. According to Borges (2017)[10] *"quality in health is to show the real concern in guaranteeing the community a service that meets their needs in all stages of health care".* In view of the above, it is clear that the understanding of quality in health will interfere in how the professional assumes his role before the community and consequently in how to provide health care in face of the specificities found.

Other research points out that, when it comes to public health, quality would be to offer greater benefits with fewer risks to as many people as possible. Its achievement would only be conceivable through compliance with minimum standards for adequate care[11] . The PMAQ-AB emerges as a tool providing subsidies for the achievement of goals and consequently the improvement of assistance to users.

Some participants associate the programme only as a financial aid provided by the government, which can be identified in the statements below:

"It is a gratification for us that is very welcome .... " (ACS2)

"I understand that it is a grant that comes to health professionals as an incentive..."(ACS1)

"[...] it is a grant that comes from the government, which is to help both in the incentive of health professionals and in the place where it is stabilized. [...] I understand that it is a grant that comes to help the health units." (ACS20)

With the creation, in 2011, of the quality component, a new way of financing the AB emerged. Adherence is voluntary and its success depends on the motivation and proactivity of all professionals of the multiprofessional team[12] .

This bonus should develop an appropriate organisational climate to influence the work process developed and thus ensure the achievement of pre-established goals benefiting those who have made the effort for such[13] .

Although the financial incentive is related to job satisfaction, this should not be highlighted as the most important and only motivational factor[14] . In a study conducted in the north of the country, the findings bring divergence of opinions among the interviewees and conclude that the forms of rewards and stimuli may be diverse and that each individual is motivated by different needs[15] .

Therefore, it is necessary that the CHAs understand the importance of the programme as a tool capable of improving the quality of care and expanding access to services, placing themselves as key agents for this transformation, since they can act directly on the particularities of each individual in the community.

PMAQ-AB: Limitations experienced by CHWs

The statements explain the difficulties encountered by CHWs in implementing the programme:

"The difficulty that we think PMAQ has, is that most of the FHPs lack structure, they work in rented houses. "(ACS21)

"...] Some things are required by PMAQ, that sometimes there is no way, right? Due to the structure, the unit here is not a PSF unit. It shouldn't be a rented house, mold, that sort of thing. "(ACS22)

Most participants mention that there is an inconsistency (theory/reality) regarding the physical structure of PHC units. Of the 17 units participating in the survey, 13 functioned in rented houses and with adaptations. According to the MS, the spaces for the maintenance of a health unit should be compatible with the local reality and should accommodate the entire population as well as its specificities. The principles of the RDC No. 50/Anvisa/2002 should be followed, which provides on the Technical Regulations for planning, programming and evaluation of physical projects of Health Care Establishments (EAS)[16] .

The inadequacy of the physical structure may become a barrier to the provision of quality care to the population, interfering with accessibility and may generate user resistance towards the health service, as well as embarrassment for the professional[17] .

Studies carried out in southern and northeastern Brazil pointed out that most health professionals recognize the influence of the ambience on the work process, impacting on their own well-being and on the reception of the population and consequently on the quality of care[18,19] .

According to Donabedian[20] , the structure contributes to the development of care processes, reflecting on their results and playing a central role in improving the quality of services. It is related to what he calls "stable conditions of the health services". That is, the material and human resources, the physical context, the organizational model and the instruments that involve health actions.

In addition, it was noticed that some FHS teams participating in this research had an insufficient number of CHAs. The statements show that this factor reflects directly on the quality of care provided, undermining the development of the PMAQ-AB:

"Well, the PMAQ it is a programme for the whole team, if the team is understaffed you can't beat targets..." (ACS7)

"Look, I think there are many difficulties, mainly in terms of personnel, which we don't have. If there was a whole team, each one would do their own job, even so, everyone ends up helping each other. "(CHW6)

According to Ordinance No. 703 of 21 October 2011, the minimum number of professionals for a FHS team should be: one nurse, one nursing assistant and one doctor, responsible for a coverage area of up to 4,000 people. It is imperative that the number of CHAs cover 100% of the registered population, with a maximum of 750 people for each in a total of 12 professionals per team[21] .

The lack of members in a minimum team brings losses related to the minimization of the offer of essential services to the health of the population, besides not receiving the ideal funding to meet the needs of users, resulting in the underutilization of materials and the impossibility of offering adequate assistance to users[13] .

In a study conducted in the north of the state of Minas Gerais using data from the PMAQ-AB self-evaluation, the quality standard "professional composition" was analyzed and it was concluded that the teams that had a greater number of professionals resulted in better classification, thus showing how impactful the lack of professionals in health services is[22] .

The literature points out that in addition to the work overload generated by the low number of professionals in the area covered by the FHS, the lack of tools to perform actions generates dissatisfaction, insecurity and a sense of loss of meaning[23] . Unfortunately, it is common that the worker working in the PCU faces scarcity of resources and technologies. However, it is known that it is necessary to have the minimum quantity required for effective results .[24]

The participants of this study also pointed out the lack of material resources as a hindering factor for the implementation and realization of the PMAQ-AB, as presented below:

"[...].lack of dressing materials, medicines, the service is very demanding, goals that you have to meet and when it is time to provide support, for example: blank sheet of paper, you have to keep asking. Folder to put files, you don't have [...]" (CHW16)

"Everything is missing here! We lack a lot of material, we have no material to work with [...]" (ACS38)

Material resources provide support to the service, ensuring that the service is provided in an effective manner. Their scarcity compromises the execution of actions and the achievement of the stipulated goals, compromising the resolubility of the service offered. It is a factor that makes the continuity of care impossible, generating dissatisfaction of the team before the working conditions offered[25] .

Potentialities of PMAQ-AB from the perspective of CHWs

The participants highlight the increase in motivation, improvement in the organization of the work process and professional qualification as potentialities arising from adhesion to the program:

"It's an incentive for us, it's a way for us to feel valued. "(CHW1)

"The benefits that the programme brought us? Well, it only increased even more the motivation for us to work...but like this, it increased the goal, but it encouraged us to work harder. "(ACS11)

"[...]the PSF welcomes differently than before. The number of attendance has improved. "(ACS30)

"The benefit that the programme brings? Ah, I think that everything organized is better, right? Things that are more organized get easier (laughs)". (ACS29)

"[...] besides you always having to be organised it ends up giving us an incentive, because there you know you will be more charged and you end up being more regulated, you end up being more certain". (ACS39)

"[...] brought many updates, we started to do things the right way, to better serve the population. "(ACS31)

"When we started we took a lot of courses, we took a lot of courses to learn how to fill out the forms, how to approach the patient..." (ACS9)

One of the programme's commitments is for municipal managers to carry out continuing education (PE) activities with the primary care teams. It is an important strategy for collective training, and a powerful resource for in-service training. Furthermore, it aims, through the problematisation of reality, to bring about changes in workers' practices, discussed and agreed in the PE group, through the definition of minimum competencies to be developed by them, necessary for the development of the practices recommended by the MS[26] .

The BS is present in all phases and sub-phases of the PMAQ-AB. Through it, there is the promotion of debates on professional development, the resolution capacity arising from the PCU, management and community participation, in addition to the articulation with the needs presented by health services according to the specificities of each territory. These issues are intertwined in order to change the practices of doing, work and service offered in order to solve the problems of the community[27] .

The process of work management requires new ways of thinking and acting towards workers' demands. It can be considered that the health sector is a living and dynamic process, which involves the encounter between two worlds, the user's world and the worker's world. This dynamic requires continuous learning processes, with actions that trigger and awaken in the workers always new processes in the making of health[27] .

CONCLUSIONS

This study showed the importance of CHWs' perception of the program and its impact on care, since the statements showed a fragmented definition of the PMAQ-AB. Still, there was an association with the financial incentive provided, being pointed out by the CHWs as a motivating element. In addition, the encouragement to professional qualification and the incorporation of the BS in the service routine were highlighted as positive aspects arising from the program.

Moreover, limitations were identified about the physical structure of the units, the insufficient number of professionals and shortage of material resources needed to carry out the actions, generating consequences in the assistance offered to the population.

Inserted in the community, CHWs integrate popular and scientific knowledge, contributing to the promotion of educational actions that reflect on the quality of health care. Despite being a relevant professional class in the context of PHC, there are still few studies that point to its influence on the quality of health. It is assumed that there will be greater awareness in the next evaluations with greater recognition of the importance of these professionals in the implementation of PMAQ-AB. Because of this, it is suggested the continuity of research on the subject.

REFERENCES

1. Silva MM, Budó MLD, Resta DG, et al. Integrality in family health: limits and possibilities from the team's perspective. Cienc Cuid Saude 2013jan/mar; 12(1):155-163.

2. Pinto HA, Sousa ANA, Ferla AA. The National Program for Improvement of Access and Quality of Basic Care: several faces of an innovative policy. Saúde debate 2014 oct;38(n.spe):358-372.

3. Cardoso AS, Nascimento MC. Communication in the Family Health Program: the health agent as an integrating link between the team and the community. Ciência & Saúde Coletiva 2010 jan;15(1):1509-20. Pedraza DF, Santos IS. Evaluation of growth surveillance in childcare consultations in the Family Health Strategy in two municipalities of the state of Paraíba, Brazil. Epidemiol. Serv. Saúde 2017 dec; 26 (4):847-855.

4. Pedraza DF, Santos IS. Evaluation of growth surveillance in childcare consultations in the Family Health Strategy in two municipalities of the state of Paraíba, Brazil. Epidemiol. Serv. Saúde 2017 dec;26(4):847-855

5. Brazil. Ministério da Saúde. Ordinance No. 1.654, of July 19, 2011. Institui, no âmbito do Sistema Único de Saúde, o Programa Nacional de Melhoria do Acesso e da Qualidade da Atenção Básica (PMAQ-AB) e o Incentivo Financeiro do PMAQ-AB, denominado Componente de Qualidade do Piso de Atenção Básica Variável - PAB Variável. Official Gazette of the Union.

6. Sampaio J, Moraes MN, Marcolino EC, et al. PMAQ-AB: the local experience for the qualification of the national program. Rev enferm UFPE on line 2016 nov; 10(Supl.5):4318-28.

7. Fonseca AF, Mendonça MHM. A interação entre avaliação e a atuação dos Agentes Comunitários de Saúde: subsídios para pensar sobre o trabalho educativo. Saude Debate 2014 oct; 38(spe):343-357.

8. Minayo MCS. The challenge of knowledge: qualitative health research. 12º Ed. São Paulo-Rio de Janeiro: HUCITEC-ABRASCO, 2010.

9. Bardin L. Content Analysis. São Paulo: Edições 70, 2011.

10. *Borges AMM, Duarte MMP, Coelho WG, et al. Quality assessment in health services: an*

integrative review. Health Care Network Journal 2017;10(1).

11. Barroso LMM, Victor JF. Qualidade dos serviços ao cliente e dos serviços de apoio em Unidade Básica da Família. Rev. RENE 2003 jan-jun; 4(1):24-29.

12. Brazil. Ministério da Saúde. Acesso e Qualidade Programa Nacional de Melhoria do Acesso e da Qualidade da Atenção Básica (PMAQ-AB). Rio de Janeiro (DF): The Ministry, 2012b.

13. Slomochenski LA. Análise do Impacto Motivacional do PMAQ-AB em relação aos Servidores Públicos da Secretaria Municipal de Santo Amaro da Imperatriz-SC [thesis] [internet] Coleção Gestão da Saúde Pública; 2013. 21p.

14. Cunha GT, Castro PC, Oliveira MM, et al. National Program to Improve Access and Quality of Primary Care: a qualitative study.In: 2° Congresso Brasileiro de política, planejamento e gestão em saúde. 2013, Belo Horizonte

15. Feitosa RMM, Paulino AA, Júnior JOSL, et al . Changes offered by the National Program for Improving Access and Quality of Primary Care. Saude soc 2016set;25(3):821-829.

16. Brazil. Ministério da Saúde. Manual de estrutura física das unidades básicas de saúde: saúde da família. 2. ed. Brasil: Ministério da Saúde, 2008 (Série A. Normas e Manuais Técnicos).

17. Pedrosa ICF, Correa ACP, Mandu ENT. Influências da infraestrutura de centros de saúde nas práticas profissionais: percepções de enfermeiros. Cienc. Cuid. Saude 2011 jan/mar;10(1).

18. Glanzn CH, Olschowsky A. Ambience and its infl uence on the work of family health teams. Health and Human Development Journal 2017 feb;5(1):7-14.

19. Oliveira MM, Pinto IC, Cruz VD, et al.Análise da estrutura de uma unidade de saúde da família sob a perspectiva da ambiência. Rev. APS 2014 oct/dec;17(4): 423-428.

20. Donabedian A, Wheeler HRC, Wysze-Wianski L. Quality, Cost, and Health: An Integrative Model. *Med. Care* 20(10): 1975-92, 1982.

21. Brazil. Ministério da Saúde. Portaria n° 703, de 21 de outubro de 2011. Institui, no âmbito do Sistema Único de Saúde, o Programa Nacional de Melhoria do Acesso e da Qualidade da Atenção Básica (PMAQ-AB) e o Incentivo Financeiro do PMAQ-AB, denominado Componente de Qualidade do Piso de Atenção Básica Variável - PAB Variável. Official Gazette of the Union.

22. Moreira KS, Vieira MA, Costa SM. Qualidade da Atenção Básica: avaliação das Equipes de Saúde da Família. Saúde debate 2016 oct-dez;40 (111).

23. Krug SBF, Santos AC, Dutra BD et al. Suffering and falling ill in the work of community health workers: a study in family health strategies. Revista UNIABEU Belford Roxo 2015 sep-dez;8(20).

24. Bender KG, Santos AC, Dutra BD et al. Conditions and modifications in the work process: conceptions of community health agents. Revista Jovens Pesquisadores, Santa Cruz do Sul 2016;6(2): 45-49.

25. Pedrosa ICF, Corrêa ACP, Mandu ENT. Influências da infraestrutura de centros de saúde nas práticas profissionais: percepções de enfermeiros. Cienc. Cuid. Saude. 2011;10(1).

26. Silva DLS, Knobloch, F. A equipe enquanto lugar de formação: a educação permanente em um Centro de Atenção Psicossocial Álcool e outras drogas. Interface (Botucatu)2016;20(57).

27. Ribeiro DT, Nascimento DT do, Cunha FM da et al. The PMAQ-AB as one of the strategies to stimulate the practice of Continuing Education in Health. Revista Saúde e Desenvolvimento Humano 2016;129-141.

CHAPTER 3

THE PROCESS OF HOSPITAL ACCREDITATION IN BRAZIL: a reflection*

*Text extracted from the Master's Dissertation "Singularities of managerial work in an Accredited hospital. UFMG Nursing School. 2012

Andréia Guerra Siman

Maria José Menezes Brito

Over time, new demands have been required and mobilised by managers, modifying their work and their performance. Faced with the option of adhering to the AH process, aiming at certification by an accrediting organization, the organizations are becoming more flexible and, above all, facing the challenge of offering answers to organizational changes, seeking assistance containing optimal quality standards. The health organization was one of the last social organizations to adopt quality management methods and models for "accreditation".

Accreditation is a tool to measure and compare health units, nationally or internationally, and offers paths of adequacy to the demand of the consuming public. The proposed process is permanent educational, involving all the actors in the health institution scenario: manager, worker and client[1,2]

.

Accreditation is a flexible process, as it allows for adaptations to the size and complexity of the organisation, which will act to the point of adapting itself, including to demands regarding the client's rights. In this context, the work process has been undergoing changes in several dimensions. Such dimensions are directly related not only to administrative actions, but also to care actions, as they involve improvements in the work process in the managerial and care aspects, with a view to providing assistance of quality and excellence. It is through managerial work that the quality of care, excellence, improvement in care focused on customer satisfaction and accreditation in health services are sought[3].

It becomes necessary to clarify the terms: "certification", "accreditation" and "quality". "Quality" is the degree to which services provided to the patient increase the likelihood of favourable outcomes. The term "certification" is used when it is a process by which a government agency or professional association officially recognizes an entity or individual as having met certain predetermined qualifications. The term "accreditation" is used for the procedure of evaluation of institutional resources; voluntary, periodic and reserved, which tends to guarantee the quality of care through previously accepted standards. The standards may be minimal or more demanding, defining different levels of satisfaction[4] .

In this book, the term accreditation used is better defined by Cordeiro (2000), in the context of health organizations, it means: [...] assessment of the conformity of the health work process with standards, that is, with statements of maximum desirable expectations of performance of a health organization (hospital, outpatient clinic, clinical analysis laboratory and other services[5] . It can be stated that the term believe reflects on quality. One cannot achieve a good performance within an organization without working on quality.

The term quality was coined in the industrial context by American thinkers who worked with quality. Its apogee was in the Japanese industry, in the post-war period. In order to transpose this quality model in the American and Japanese industries to the health area, Donabedian (1998) pointed out six key attributes that form the basis for quality in health: effectiveness; efficiency; balance in the costs of care provided; meeting the expectations of customers and family members; provision of care meeting ethical standards, values, standards, regulations and laws; and equity in care[6] .

In a more modern context, the term quality means continuous improvement. Quality equals satisfied customers. It translates a phenomenon that involves improvement, establishment of standards and results, performance of actions without defects and quality management. Through quality the manager is able to identify flaws in routines and procedures in a permanent review process, involving the entire body of the organisation[2] . Before the accreditation movement reached Brazil in the 1970s, the initial objective of the World Health Organization (WHO) was to provide a standard of health that would allow all individuals the opportunity to live a socially and economically productive life, the goal of "Health for All". In the 1980s, WHO set the goal of "Health for All" to be achieved by the year 2000. The concern with the quality of health care offered by institutions grew. It was in this context of renewed concern with the fulfillment of the goal pleaded for the XXI century that the theme "accreditation" has expanded in the world scenario .[3]

In 1989, adopting this comprehensive theme "The quality of care", the World Health Organization started in the hospital area in America, which became the starting point for triggering quality initiatives in health services. It was intended to evaluate aspects such as strengths and weaknesses of the institutions[7] . Since then, the quality strategy has expanded in Latin American countries. In this scenario of quality in health, the conquest for accreditation has been consolidating in Brazil. From 1988 to 1999, the Ministry of Health carried out several projects in an attempt to implement a methodology for evaluating the quality of care.

To improve the quality in health in Brazil, after the 1980s, with the physician Humberto Moraes Novaes in the coordination of the Pan-American Health Organization, hospital standards were established in Latin America for hospitals to reach and receive the condition of "accredited", creating improvements in health services. It was also an initiative in the development of methodologies to reach hospital accreditation[8] . In 1992, in Brasilia, according to Feldman and Cunha[2] , the project of disclosure of AH was carried out, with cycles of lectures in locations in the national sphere, reaching all regions of the country. The objective was to present the project for a better understanding of the accreditation system, which culminated in the creation of the entity National Accreditation Organization (ONA).

In Brazil, this expansion was possible due to the publication of "Accreditation of Hospitals for Latin America and the Caribbean", which then, together with the Ministry of Health (MS) in 1995, presented the Brazilian Program of Quality and Productivity, for the implementation of Hospital Accreditation (AH) (BRASIL, 2006). The intention of the MS was to provide an overview of the rationality, activities, tools, technologies and structures that characterize the quality assurance, its development and accreditation in health .[3]

The ONA was created in 1999, concretizing and expanding the inclusion of hospitals in the accreditation process. In 2001, the MS suggested that participation of health institutions in the process of AH as voluntary and considered as part of public policy the adoption of methodologies to guarantee the quality of care in Brazilian hospitals, by Administrative Rule 538, of 14/04/2001[9] . ANVISA (2004) officially recognized the Brazilian Accreditation System in 2002, by Resolution 921/02. To further integrate the National System of Health Surveillance, the Agency included in the programming of the agreement the free course of distance learning, via internet "Evaluation of Health Services, Health Licensing and Accreditation", directed to the state and municipal Health Surveillance, to professionals of health services and managers of the Unified Health System (SUS)[8]
.

In relation to the ONA, it is a private, non-profit and collective interest organization, with the objective of implanting and implementing, on a national level, a permanent process to improve the quality of health care, influencing all health services in the AH process. With the strong discussion on quality in health and the competitive market among hospital institutions, in 1999, the Hospital Israelita Albert Einstein was the first in the world to be internationally accredited, earning the International Accreditation Certificate, a milestone. From then on, changes were observed in the standards of care and service provision, initially within the hospitals in downtown São Paulo[2,8] .

According to data from the Global Review, by the year 2003, 123 health services (56 hospitals) were accredited worldwide, including Brazil. The International Manual of Standards for Hospital Accreditation pointed out that 40 hospitals were accredited by the Joint Commission on Accreditation of Hospitals (JCAH) methodology in the world. This data has been growing every year. With the methodology of the National Accreditation Organization (ONA), the Organization disclosed that only in Minas Gerais until May 2018 43 were accredited[11] .

The accreditation is one of the evaluation methods of health organizations that indicate measures for the continuous improvement of the quality of care provided by Brazilian hospitals, regardless of their size, complexity, and institutional affiliation. Considering Ordinance GM/MS 538, dated April 17, 2001[9] , the ONA was recognized as a competent and authorized institution to operate the development of the hospital accreditation process. The ONA defines the accreditation process as a method of consensus, rationalization and ordering of the Hospital Service Provider Organizations and, especially, of the continuing education of its professionals.

The ONA is a regulatory and accrediting body for the development of quality improvement in health. Its manual has descriptions of standards that certify and propose quality levels to be achieved. It is the Brazilian Manual of Hospital Accreditation (MBAH)[2] . According to ONA, the MBAH is a specific instrument to assess the quality of care in these institutions systemically and globally. It is an instrument to define norms and assess whether the service meets previously established standards regarding the quality of care. Approval of the MBAH is the responsibility of the Ministry of Health. It needs to be periodically revised and adapted to the reality of Brazilian hospitals, in order to improve the process of hospital accreditation in the country[10] .

To enable the achievement of quality standards, in 1998, the first publication of the Brazilian Manual of Hospital Accreditation (MBAH) was launched[10] , which had two functions: to expose a flexible scheme to provide the incorporation of the hospital in the network of services; and to give direction for the development of the quality of services[3] . In 2010, ONA presented its first edition of the MBAH of Health Programs and Risk Prevention[12] . The manuals published and ONA are a way to enable self-evaluation and constant improvement of the quality provided as a whole. It is a way of ordering health organizations, of continuing education for managers and their staff.

In order to achieve accredited status, the health care organization undergoes a process that requires the following requirements: to be voluntary, to follow the assessment manual, to perform an external verification by an accrediting institution accredited by the ONA[13] . For ANVISA (2004), to be accredited, the health establishment must undergo this assessment, made by an independent organization, accredited by the ONA, receiving a preliminary diagnosis. At the end of the process, it must meet the quality standards defined in the diagnosis for each work area. The initial diagnosis may be considered the starting point of the process, "it may be compared to an x-ray of the organisation's operation and serves as a basis to propose changes"[8:335] ; and a master plan will be established to guide the necessary changes. The diagnostic visit has the function of assessing and certifying the institution based on the standards and norms defined at national level, standards which were elaborated in three levels, correlated and of increasing complexity.

The accreditation process according to ONA[12] is structured in three levels. Level 1) "Accredited" - requests basic requirements of quality in the assistance and has as principle the safety of the patient in all areas of activity, including structural and assistance aspects. It contemplates quality care provided to the patient with professional qualifications and specialties compatible with the complexity of the service. Requires planning in the organization of hospital care. Contemplates the verification of documentation and the staff, worker training, routines and indicators for decision making, with a clinical and managerial action plan, in addition to the internal audit practice. Level 3) "Accredited with Excellence" - principle based on management excellence (results). It is based on continuous improvements in the structures, in the technical professional updating, in new technologies, in assistance actions with standardized and evaluated routines, and in medical-sanitary procedures, aiming at reaching the excellence[10] .

Once approved, the health organisation receives the Accredited Organisation Certificate, which is valid for two years for Levels 1 and 2, and three years for Level 3. The organisations are submitted to a new evaluation at the end of this period to maintain and ensure the quality standard. The process is concluded with the issuance of the report by the accreditation commission and the delivery of the final opinion to the organisation providing health services. With the qualification, benefits are achieved in the health-disease process, including the capacity to transmit greater safety to the patient and greater personal security.

For the provision of quality health services, elements such as humanization, communication between those involved, compliance with the patient's right to information and continuing education are essential. In this process, the bond between professionals, patients and workers interferes with quality, as a significant relationship of trust between them is necessary throughout the care process. It is worth noting that customers have concrete and particular needs and that health organizations need to meet this demand in the best possible way, according to the reality in which it is inserted.

The responsibility of accredited hospitals goes beyond the concern to maintain certification. They may emerge as an example of management of their services and as a model for other health organizations that want, as a built external image, safety, quality, efficiency, effectiveness and ethics. To integrate the accreditation is an option of the health institution, but it has a great responsibility before society, which imposes the maintenance of quality standards during the assistance to internal and external customers.

In this sense, it is worth noting that it is necessary to treat accreditation without getting carried away by the passionate movement of thinking of quality only as ideology[3] . Accreditation demands from the manager and all actors involved a continuous commitment to maintain quality, performing their actions within the established standards of excellence and not only achieving the certification but maintaining it, building a culture of quality.

Adoption of quality systems: perspectives of the health sector. The health services sector, unlike productive sectors such as industry, has not yet built a tradition of adopting quality management systems. Everything is relatively new, but the trend in this sector is to seek to adopt quality assurance systems. The concern with quality comes from the industrial context, in which the main focus was to elaborate quality control methods[14] .

Mezomo[15] addresses the concept of quality based on the perspective of the importance of customer satisfaction with the services offered. In this sense, quality means "conformity to requirements", relating quality to a standard, which, once defined, initiates high quality production. It is doing the right thing the first time and better the next. The quality management models of general use in healthcare in Brazil are: the National Accreditation Organization (ONA) or International Canadian Council on Health Services Accreditation (CCHSA), Joint Commission International (JCI) and National Integrated Accreditation for Healthcare Organizations (NIAHO).

However, some organizations adopt ABNT NBR ISSO 9001 to establish their quality management system[14]. The accreditation of health organizations presents itself as a way to improve service management, and not only as a mere certification, due to the impact on the management of quality care, considering that, by meeting the quality standards, it stimulates the consolidation and construction of management and quality assurance[14].

With the adoption of the quality policy in health services, the perspective is that it effectively contributes to the development of quality in all senses, reaching the satisfaction of internal customers (professionals) and external (patients) and establishing continuous improvement of its processes and results.

SEARCH FOR QUALITY: THE HOSPITAL AND ITS INSERTION IN THE HEALTH CARE NETWORK

In order to approach the quality of health services, involving the fulfillment of the health needs and demands of the population and the provision of better services in hospital care, it is indispensable to discuss the hospital and its insertion in the health care network. This is because the process of hospital accreditation and its quality policy, according to Novaes[1] is directly related to the development of countries, notably as to education and culture, and with the recognition of citizens of their rights to quality health care.

The definition of the World Health Organization (WHO) fits here: The hospital is an integral part of a coordinated health system, whose function is to provide the community with complete health care, both curative and preventive, including services extended to the family at home, and also a training centre for those working in the health field and for biosocial research (16: 122).

.

Hospitals have a privilege in health and social policies because, even if the municipality has Basic Units and Outpatient Clinics, the care model ignores the need for integration of actions and integrality of care[17]. Thus, hospitals need to have new working models, in view of the changes generated nowadays. Such changes are of epidemiological, demographic, cultural, technological and economic nature, and have been transforming the models of health care and, consequently, implying transformations in the hospital network[17].

With regard to changes, in the 20th century Brazil experienced intense transformations in its population structure and in the morbidity and mortality pattern. In relation to epidemiological changes, the decrease in general mortality, the continuous increase in life expectancy at birth and the reduction of birth rates and population growth are highlighted. As a consequence, there is an increase in the group of people aged 65 years or more, generating impacts on the consumption of health services, since this age group has greater demand in hospital admissions[17,18] .

With regard to demographic changes, the decrease in infectious and parasitic diseases and the increase in diseases and mortalities from chronic diseases and non-communicable diseases, such as cardiovascular diseases and neoplasms, and external causes[17,18] stand out. The return of diseases such as tuberculosis, dengue and cholera, called re-emerging diseases, reveal a picture potentiated by the emergence of emerging infectious-contagious diseases such as AIDS, hantavirus, human spongiform disease, and the growing resistance of bacteria to antibiotics, and social problems such as violence, accidents, alcoholism, smoking and other drugs with repercussions on morbidity and mortality[17,18] .

This context has repercussions on the demand and use of care actions that accompany the real health needs of the population. The specialization and technological development have also intensely affected the hospital organization, which has acquired greater ability to diagnose, although with uncontrolled increase in spending, without cost-benefit criteria in the incorporation of an original Text in Spanish technologies[19] . This set of changes causes several alterations, which involve from work practices, changes in management and changes in the distribution of resources (people and their competences), to changes in the operating rules, as well as in the relationships between the other components of the health system[18] .

For the survival and the achievement of the objectives for which they were created, the organizations do not need and cannot be self-sufficient. Hospital organisations need inter-relationships, cooperation, complementarity among other organisations and flexible structures capable of establishing vertical and horizontal relationships, thus achieving the organisation's purpose, which is to provide a quality service[18] .

For an approach to the hospital network, it is worth highlighting the concept of health care networks, which, according to Mendes[19] , are conceptualized as polyarchic organizations of sets of health services linked together by a single mission, by common objectives and by a cooperative and interdependent action that allows offering continuous and comprehensive health care to a given population. Thus, the provision of health services should not be organized in rigid and segmented levels of care, but in networks that include hospitals as active members with the various actors and public, private, philanthropic entities or various components of the system.

Since its creation, the hospital has undergone modifications. The hospital was created to isolate people with infectious diseases from society. Today it is an organisation aimed at solving the health problems of the community in which it is located. The hospital was based on a historical, biomedical and curative model of care, with a culture predominantly of self-sufficiency, together with the medical professional. An organisation seen with more power, with a modulating and hegemonic role in the health system[18].

Therefore, the hospital in the context of a health care network breaks the paradigm in which it was the only entity providing health care services and breaks with the position of central axis of the health system. Currently, in the health care model, according to several authors[10,18,21], the axis, the gateway and the regulatory centre of the health care network is Primary Health Care (PHC). In this context, the MH, among other public providers, is increasingly aware of the need to conceive hospitals as members of the network of public and private services. In this sense, effectiveness is fundamental, which includes appropriate information management systems, communication and referral and counter-referral of patients, which requires a level of relationship between hospitals and Primary Care establishments .[18]

The challenge that many countries begin to face is to articulate service networks (public and private, community and decentralized) that overcome the bureaucratic and hierarchical management; the dividing line between promotion, prevention, cure and rehabilitation activities, the management barriers between primary and specialized, increasing the resolution capacity, articulating public and private providers, ensuring the continuity of care[18: 81]. This system, established in a well organized network, has the possibility to bring several benefits, such as: resolubility, better coverage and ease of access, less consumption of resources, more efficiency and continuity of care with higher quality and with more satisfied patients and families.

According to PAHO, the essential thing is the political decision to set up a network service provision that integrates the different services to ensure the optimization of resources and comprehensive and resolute care to the health needs of users[18]. However, the challenge of ensuring universal access, with comprehensive care, in an efficient, hierarchical and regionalized manner, is more directed to the public sector than to the private. One of the additional problems facing this situation is management. All municipalities in Brazilian cities, even those with less than 10,000 inhabitants, want to have their own hospital. In truth, the small municipalities should have guaranteed access in the network, and the success of this is the hierarchization of the network, in addition to the effectiveness of the computerization of the systems.

Thus, it would contribute so that all citizens have access to all kinds of services[17]. The relationship between public hospitals and private hospitals passes through a discussion between the public manager, society and the Public Ministry. One of the steps to this challenge is to keep private care as complementary, being fundamental to set up the network of regulation and seek to transform the difficulty of access faced in a transparent and accountable way to society[17] .

REFERENCES

1-NOVAES, H. M. O processo de acreditação dos serviços de saúde. Revista de Administração e Saúde, v.9, n.37, out-dez. 2007.

2- FELDMAN, L.B.; GATTO, M.A.F; CUNHA, I.C.K.O. História da evolução da qualidade hospitalar: dos padrões a acreditarão. Acta Paul Enferm, São Paulo, n. 18, p. 213-219. 2005

3- FORTES, M. T. R et al. The accreditation or accreditations? A comparative study between accreditation in France, the United Kingdom and Catalonia. Rev Assoc Med Bras, Rio de Janeiro, v. 57, n. 2, p. 239-246. 2011.

4- BITTAR, O.J.N.V. Cultura e qualidade em hospitais. In: QUINTO NETO, A.; BITAR, O.J.N.V. Hospitais: adminstração da qualidade e acreditação de organizações complexas. Porto Alegre: Da Casa; 2004. 17 p.

5- CORDEIRO, H. Acreditação de Serviços de Saúde: Controversies, Perspectivas e Tendências para o Melhororamento da Qualidade. In: CORDEIRO, H. ENSAIO: Avaliação e Políticas em Educação. Rio de Janeiro: Cesgranrio Foundation, Special Number, v. 8, June, 2000.

6- DONABEDIAN, A. The quality of health: how can not be assured? JAMA, v. 260, p. 1743-1748. 1998.

7- KISIL, M.; SCHIESARI L. M. C. Avaliação da qualidade nos hospitais brasileiros. RAS vol. 5, n 18, Jan-Mar, 2003.

8- ANVISA- National Health Surveillance Agency. Acreditação: a busca pela qualidade nos serviços de saúde. Rev Saúde Pública, v. 38, n.2. p. 335-336. 2004.

9- BRAZIL. Ministry of Health. PORTARIA N° 538, DE 17 DE ABRIL DE 2001.

10- BRAZIL. Ministry of Health. Secretariat of Health Assistance. Department of care networks. Manual Brasileiro de Acreditação Hospitalar. 7.ed. Brasília: Ministry of Health, 2006.

11- -NATIONAL ACCREDITATION ORGANIZATION (ONA). Meet the ONA. 2018.Available at:<https://www.ona.org.br/Pagina/20/Conheca-a-ONA>.

12- BRASIL. National Accreditation Organization. Manual de Organizações Prestadoras de Serviços Hospitalares. Brasília: ONA, 2010.

13- LABBADIA, L. L.; et al. O processo de Acreditação Hospitalar e a participação da enfermeira. Rev Enferm UERJ, Rio de Janeiro, v. 12, n.1, p.83-87, abr. 2004.

14- KERN, A. E; LIMA, A. P. F. O gestor da área de qualidade. In: ALVES, V.L.S. FELDMAN, L.B. Gestores da saúde no âmbito da qualidade: atuação e competências abordagem multidisciplinar. 1. ed. São Paulo: Martinari, 2011.

15- MEZOMO, J. C. Gestão da qualidade na saúde: princípios básicos. 1. ed. São Paulo: Loyola,

2001. 301 p.

16- WORLD HEALTH ORGANIZATION. Committee of Experts on Organization of Medical Care. Función de los hospitales en los programas de protección de la salud. Ver Inform. Tecn, v 4, n 122, 1957.

17- VECINA, G. NETO; MALIK, A. M. Tendências na assistência hospitalar. Ciência e Saúde Coletiva, v. 12, n. 4, p. 825-839, 2007.

18- PAHO- Pan American Health Organization. The transformation of hospital management in Latin America and the Caribbean. Brasília: PAHO/WHO, 2004. 389 p.

19- CECÍLIO, L.C.O; FEUERWERKER, L.C.M. O hospital e a formação em saúde: desafios atuais. Ciência & Saúde Coletiva, n.12, v.4, p.965-971. 2007.

20- MENDES, EV. Health care networks. Revista Médica de Minas Gerais (RMMG). MG, v. 18, n. 4-S4, 2008.

21- CECILIO, L. C. O. Modelos tecno-assistenciais em saúde: da pirâmide ao círculo, uma possibilidade a ser explorada. Cad. Saúde Pública, Rio de Janeiro, v. 13, n. 3, Sept. 1997.

CHAPTER 4

HOSPITAL ACCREDITATION: THE EXPERIENCE OF IMPLEMENTATION IN A TEACHING HOSPITAL

Marilane de Oliveira Fani Amaro
Andréia Guerra Siman Camilo
Amaro de Carvalho Gabriela
Rezende Moreira Neiva

INTRODUCTION

The new managerial models, competitiveness and the search for quality in the health area have triggered expressive changes in the hospital environment and in health institutions. More and more, citizens understand quality as a social right, demanding it from health services, resulting in excellence in the environments providing such services[1] .

Quality is understood as an attribute of the service, it should be in accordance with the mission of the organisation and should aim to provide adequate response to the needs and expectations of the user. Thus, it can be observed through customer satisfaction and obtained through the efficient use of available resources, in addition to professional qualification. Furthermore, its maintenance is provided by the joint work of users, professionals and managers[2] .

The lack of quality in health services impacts professionals, patients and society, resulting in rework; ineffective services, which do not achieve the expected results; inefficient services, with high costs; and inaccessible services, which reflect in the dissatisfaction of users and health professionals[3] .

As of the 1990s, models of external evaluation of health services emerged in Brazil, such as hospital accreditation, for quality assessment in hospitals. Currently, there are different hospital accreditation models in our country: National Accreditation Organization (ONA); *Joint Commission International* (JCI); Canadian *Accreditation; National Integrated Accreditation for Healthcare Organizations* (NIAHO); certification by ISO 9.001, 14.000, 31.000 and OHSAS 18.001 standards[4] .

In Brazil, 242 hospitals are certified by the ONA methodology. In Minas Gerais, 40 are accredited, but the Zona da Mata Mineira has only four accredited hospital institutions[5] . Thus, the concern with the assessment of health services and quality in hospitals located in the interior of Minas Gerais, which represents only 10% of the accredited institutions in the state, is highlighted[6] .

The Hospital Accreditation Process (PAH) is a method of periodic evaluation of the quality and provision of care, with continuous improvements and standards to be followed, focused on continuing education projects that enable changes in internal and external processes of the organization[7] .

The PAH in Brazil is a voluntary and periodic assessment system. Certification by ONA can be done in three levels: safety (level 1), integrated management (level 2) and excellence in management (level 3). In relation to level 1, the institution is evaluated focusing on patient safety, guaranteed by maintenance of the physical structure, human resources and materials, work processes and quality of records. As to level 2, assistance and interaction among all processes involved in care are analysed. Finally, level 3 assessment covers the use of information for decision making and the results and impact of interventions on the population served are analysed. The accredited institutions use the Brazilian Manual of Hospital Accreditation (MBAH) as methodological basis and the assessment is carried out by institutions accredited by the ONA, the Accrediting Institutions (IAC)[8] .

Nursing is an area of knowledge capable of performing care, administrative, educational and research activities. Therefore, it can stimulate changes in the organizational environment and improve the work process, achieving customer satisfaction. They are essential professionals for the execution of the PAH, being important in the maintenance of its actions[2] . Moreover, the nursing team represents almost 60% of the health team and is present 24 hours a day in hospital institutions, enabling greater understanding of the work process and greater stimulus to the adherence of the other team professionals to the PAH[6] . In this context, nursing management performed in the various sectors of health institutions becomes essential for the achievement of excellence, for its ability to obtain results.

Given the importance of nurses' involvement in achieving hospital accreditation and the relevance of this professional's understanding of the process for its continuity, this study was conducted to understand the meaning of the PAH for nurses from a teaching hospital located in the Zona da Mata Mineira that wishes to achieve ONA certification.

Given the above, the guiding questions of this study are: What is the importance of the HAP for nurses in a hospital institution and what are the barriers that hinder the implementation of this process?

Thus, it aimed to understand, from the nurses' perspective, the importance of the PAH and the barriers that hinder the implementation of this process.

METHODS
This is a descriptive study, qualitative in nature. Qualitative research is concerned with a reality that cannot be quantified and may answer subjective questions involving meanings, motives, beliefs and attitudes[9] .

The study scenario was a hospital located in Zona da Mata Mineira, Brazil, accredited as a teaching hospital. The choice for this location was due to being a teaching institution, linked to a university in the region, which wishes to achieve quality certification by the ONA methodology.

The population was composed of all nurses of the institution: 24 participants. Inclusion criteria were nurses who worked in the institution and exclusion criteria were those who were away from their job for any reason.

Data collection occurred in August and September 2014, through an interview with a semi-structured script containing the following guiding questions: What do you understand by Hospital Accreditation Process? What is the importance of this process? What actions do you need to develop for the institution to achieve Accreditation? What difficulties have you faced in this process? What is the role of nursing in the Accreditation Process?

The interviews were recorded to ensure the reliability of the data and transcribed in full for further analysis. The evaluation was performed by the Content Analysis technique, by Lawrence Bardin, who suggests sequence of analysis based on the following chronological steps: pre-analysis, material exploration, treatment of results and interpretation[10] . Initially, exhaustive reading of the answers was carried out for familiarization with the text and understanding of the meaning that the participant was trying to convey. Next, thematic classification was carried out with identification of nuclei of meaning. To ensure the anonymity of the subjects, the interviews were numbered according to the sequence in which they occurred.

The research was approved by the Ethics Committee on Research with Human Beings of the Federal University of Viçosa, through CAAE No. 30426414.8.0000.5153. The ethical precepts for the study followed resolution 466/12 of the National Health Council, which supported the preparation and signing of the Informed Consent Form. Prior authorization to conduct the study was requested to the Board of Directors of the hospital where the research took place, receiving a favorable opinion from the Research Ethics Committee of the institution.

RESULTS AND DISCUSSION

Twenty-four nurses participated in the study, 71% were female. Regarding the time of graduation of the interviewees, 42% exercised the profession in the period of one to five years; 21%, six to ten years; and 37%, more than ten years. Regarding Post-Graduation, 75% of the participants specialized in areas such as Teaching, Urgency and Emergency, Cardiology and Hemodynamics, Adult and Neonatal Intensive Care, Hospital Administration, Management and Hospital Administration in Public Health and Business Management.

The analysis of the statements allowed grouping the results into three thematic categories: Importance of the PAH; Barriers to implementation of the PAH and the Role of nursing in the PAH.

Importance of PAH

The HAP is still little discussed in educational institutions, reflecting directly in the field of work[2] . It was observed that many interviewees showed insecurity or unawareness when asked about the importance of the process for the health institution:

"Very little to speak the truth with you" (E1)

"[...] I can't talk [...]" (E2)

"[...] I don't know how to answer you for sure" (E15)

It is noteworthy that, regardless of the nurse's training, the existence of permanent education in the health institution becomes fundamental to obtain a cycle of continuous improvement. The implementation of the quality process implies a vision of the future, involvement of people (at all levels and obtained through a consistent education and training plan) and creation of a support structure and monitoring of the process[11] .

Regarding the category **"Importance of the PAH"**, the following constituent elements were listed: **Organization and Standardization of the Service, Quality Improvement, Evaluation of the Institution**. Participants recognize the PAH as an important tool for **Service Organization and Standardization**:

"[...] the ONA had here to evaluate the hospital and we had to improve: identify the things that were not identified, check validity, improve standard of care quality in relation to SAE [...]" (E9)

"The hospital accreditation process [...] serves to be able to organise the service, the work [...]" (I10)

"I understand that it is to be able to maintain a standard [...]" (E21)

The statements are consistent with studies that state that Hospital Accreditation promotes progressive and planned changes of habits, values and behaviours in health institutions, aiming at organising care and standardising processes, reflecting on the improvement of organisational management[1,8] .

Some interviewees believe that the PAH aims at **Quality Improvement** in customer service and in the work process, obtained by improvements in health care, in the availability of resources and in work relations:

"[...] both in the quality of the service provided and the quality [...] of service for the professionals here" (E6)

"[...] the institution seeks excellence in human resources, in materials, in technology, in assistance [...]" (E7)

"It is showing the development of the work, it is valuing" (E12)

"[...] is for us to seek the quality of the health service, promoting better care for the patient" (E14)

It is emphasized that the PAH is a tool used by health institutions to execute a process of improvement of patient care and working conditions of the professional[1,2] . The process has evidence that it promotes increments in hospital management, providing a safe, functional and operational environment for patients, families and professionals. This improvement contributes significantly to the quality of the service provided, impacting effectively on the satisfaction of the consumer and the gain of well-being .[12]

It was observed that some nurses understand the PAH as a method of **Evaluation of the Institution**, as illustrated:

"The responsible body will check whether the service is being provided with the necessary quality or not" (E3)

"I believe that it is a process where some points of the hospitals will be evaluated [...] with regard to the quality of care and that it will be classified into levels" (E6)

"The hospital will look for ways to prove an excellence in something [...] to have a title" (E7)

"It is a certification that qualifies the hospital as a hospital that is able to serve the population" (E14); "So it's like an ISO in health, it's a quality process and it is subdivided into three classes, 1, 2 and 3, and it's about quality in service provision" (E20)

"[...] I understand the accreditation process as a process of charging for improvement" (E24)

The understanding that the PAH has only an evaluative character may be a limiting aspect of its implementation. In fact, the PAH is an evaluative method of all the resources of the institution and its purpose is to ensure assistance with defined standards. However, it also has an educational nature, which encourages the formation of responsible awareness. Therefore, it is emphasized that accreditation should be understood in two dimensions: the first, as an educational process that leads institutions providing health care services and health professionals to acquire a culture of quality for the implementation of excellence management, fundamental to the process; and the second, as a process of evaluation and certification of the quality of services, analyzing and certifying the degree of performance achieved by the institution according to predefined standards[11,13] .

Barriers to implementation of the PAH

The barriers to the implementation of the HAP include **Ineffective Management** and **Scarce Resources**.

Ineffective Management is a hindering aspect for the implementation and continuity of the PAH. When there is devaluation of the process by the institution's management, the continuation of the PAH becomes difficult, favouring its discontinuity.

"Because many times this process is almost omitted by the institution. [...] So, I think that is what is missing, a firmer position by the management, so that people follow the thing" (E23)

"[...] if all the leaders, from all the sectors, do not support it, there is no way" (E14)

"[...] I think it is a very relevant theme, still little worked on and that still needs to be well, right, more publicized" (I19)

"Because nobody is talking about the accreditation process anymore. So it was kind of forgotten" (E20)

It is noteworthy that managers play a strategic role in the development of the PAH, promoting articulation between the various sectors and professionals. Therefore, they contribute to the dissemination of knowledge related to the improvements that the organisation aims to achieve, enabling greater involvement of professionals. Without support and encouragement from the institution's management, the PAH becomes difficult to reach[14] .

It is expected that the administration of the institution assumes its role in the health organisation seeking quality in the services offered to society[12] .

The **scarcity of resources** - physical, material or human - was another aspect pointed out as a notable hindrance to the implementation of the PAH in the institution.

"[...] Sometimes it will be lacking in physical area" (E2)

"[...] a lot of equipment is missing, a lot of material is missing" (E3)

"The demand for patient care here is very high and our number of staff is somewhat reduced" (E6)

"We work in a philanthropic institution, right, which is not for profit, and has a lot of depreciated material" (I12)

The institution in the research scenario is philanthropic. Such institutions are so classified by applying 20% of annual gross revenue in gratuity; providing 60% of total admissions to the Unified Health System (SUS); or being considered strategic hospital for SUS. It is known that investment in the public network is low, representing only 3.5% of the country's Gross Domestic Product. In addition, resources are poorly managed and the administrative and operational processes are outdated and high-cost. Such facts reflect in lack of structure, reduction in the number of beds, disqualification of procedures and large debts[15] .

However, it is observed that the emphasis of accreditation does not depend only on the technological resources involved, but on the quality of the service provided. Health care should be of excellence, using the technology present in the institution. Thus, both public and private hospitals will have to adapt to the same quality standards. Aiming at improving the quality of health care offered in the institution, the PAH values the continuous and effective training of human resources, correct dimensioning of employees and continuing education of professionals involved in assistance[16] .

The role of nursing in PAH

Data analysis allowed us to identify that, in the nurses' view, the role played by nursing in the PAH is related to **Co-responsibility for Quality** and **Care Management**.

The nurse was considered an important professional for the implementation of the PAH:

"Without the nurses, they don't get the accreditation" (E4)

"If there wasn't the work of the nurse to be able to, for the hospital to be accredited, I don't think there is [...] how to do it" (E8)

The nursing team remains most of the time close to the patient, providing care from hospital admission to discharge. The individual's perception of the care they receive, together with their expectations when entering the health service, may be one of the factors that define their degree of satisfaction[17] . Nursing is capable of mobilizing the health team to solve daily problems, making the team more participative and aware in the search for quality. However, even though it occupies a fundamental place in driving this search and maintaining the accredited institution, nursing alone does not guarantee quality in care[13,14] . In this context, according to the participants, nursing has a role of **co-responsibility for Quality.** The statements reveal:

"I think it's fundamental because we are with the patient all the time. [...] like it or not, everything revolves around [...] nursing. So, I think we end up being largely responsible for the satisfaction or dissatisfaction with the service" (P3)

"...] quality, like it or not, is linked to the patient. Who has direct contact with the patient is the nursing staff" (P14)

It is emphasized that nursing is not the only professional category responsible for user satisfaction, in view of the collective work in health institutions. The quality of care requires interdisciplinary work and comprehensive care to the user, overcoming fragmented care. It becomes necessary that the various professional classes of the institution organize themselves and act together so that the user perceives the quality care[18] . The measures aimed at improving care require a broad view of the entire health team and not only nursing, so that concrete changes occur and that aim to achieve standards of care increasingly higher and consistent with the expectations of users .[17]

Care Management was also cited as a nursing role that stands out in the PAH. The unit nurse manager, in addition to implementing standards and routines, manages costs and human resources. Furthermore, he is constantly stimulated to seek innovations in the quality of care and of management itself, with the objective of producing increasingly better results. For this, he/she uses people management, sharing knowledge and transmitting information to the other components of the team[19] . The planning of actions, the organization of the environment and the systematization of techniques and procedures have also been shown as managerial roles that reflect in the execution of best practices[20] . The testimonies corroborate:

"[...] nursing [...] that will organize, so, the administrators, I think there has to be a leader in this, and he has to manage. So, nursing is a bigger team and it is us who will, [...], do more training, more organization in the sectors" (E18)

"It depends more on the administration, [...] collecting data related to the profession, [...] making a diagnosis of the sector, what it needs today, in the long and medium term" (E7)

"I think that we, as nurse coordinators, it is our obligation to pay attention to this, to medical records, to checking if the doctor is doing it or not, if the boys are correctly taking their medication

or not, if... if everything is organised or not" (I9)

"The nurse I think is one of the most important ones. Which is to seek new techniques, more appropriate techniques and guide the rest of the team to perform the correct functions" (P2)

The nurse can directly influence the quality of service by promoting the development of the nursing team and encouraging service innovation. In the operational scope, the nurse continuously and systematically supervises the nursing team according to the strategies defined to maintain the quality standard enabling the achievement of the accreditation of the health institution[18,21] .

CONCLUSION

Os resultados desta pesquisa permitem considerar que o PAH é um importante instrumento de organização do trabalho e melhoria da qualidade prestada, possibilitando avaliação das instituições hospitalares. However, part of the nurses of the institution does not understand the real meaning of the process or perceives it in a restricted way, a fact that hinders its implementation. In addition, professionals are faced with barriers that hinder the process, such as lack of resources and inefficient management.

Meanwhile, there is an urgent need to prioritize continuing education on the topic, in order to actively include professionals in the process and empower them on the subject, preventing failures related to knowledge about the PAH to compromise its implementation and continuity. It is emphasized the importance of addressing the topic in universities and other nursing education institutions, with the aim of training skilled and co-responsible professionals in relation to the quality processes of health institutions.

Regarding the limitations of the study, it is noteworthy that it was conducted in a single hospital institution and cannot express the reality of other municipalities and/or health institutions. Thus, it is suggested that further studies be conducted for greater generalization of the results.

REFERENCES

1. Manzo BF, Ribeiro HCTC, Brito MJM, Alves M. As percepções dos profissionais de saúde sobre o processo de acreditação hospitalar. Rev Enferm UERJ 2011 oct/dec;19(4):571-6.

2. Maziero VG, Spiri WC. Significance of the hospital accreditation process for nurses from a state public hospital. Rev Eletr Enf 2013;15(1):121-9.

3. Manzo BF, Ribeiro HCTC, Brito MJM, Alves M. A enfermagem no processo de acreditação hospitalar: atuação e implicações no cotidiano de trabalho. Rev Lat Am Enfermagem 2012 jan/fev;20(1).

4. Schiesari LMC. External evaluation of hospital organizations in Brazil: can we do differently? Cien Saude Colet 2014;19(10):4229-34.

5. National Accreditation Organization - ONA. Certificações válidas. São Paulo [accessed 19: Feb. 2016]. Available from: https://www.ona.org.br/OrganizacoesCertificadas.

6. Sobrinho FM, Ribeiro HCTC, Alves M, Manzo BF, Nunes SMV. Performance in the accreditation process of public hospitals of Minas Gerais/Brazil: influences for the quality of care. Enferm. Glob 2015 jan;37:298-309.

7. Manzo BF, Brito MJM, Corrêa AR. Implicações do processo de Acreditação Hospitalar no cotidiano de profissionais de saúde. Rev Esc Enferm USP 2012;46(2):388-94.

8. National Accreditation Organization. Manual of Health Service Providers Organizations. Coleção Manual Brasileiro de Acreditação. Brasília (Brazil): Organização Nacional de Acreditação; 2014.

9. Minayo MCS. The challenge of knowledge: qualitative health research. 10a ed. São Paulo: Hucitec; 2007.

10. Bardin L. Análise de conteúdo. 4ª ed. Lisboa: Edições 70; 2009. 229 p.

11. Manzo BF, Brito MJM, Correa AR. Acreditação hospitalar: aspectos dificultadores na perspectiva de profissionais de saúde de um hospital privado. REME 2011 abr/jun;15(2): 259-66.

12. Jorge MJ, de Carvalho FAA, Jorge MF, Medeiros RO. Organizational environment management in the expansion and development of the health services market in Brazil. Rev Med Minas Gerais 2012 jan/mar; 22(1): 1-128.

13. Manzo BF, Ribeiro HCTC, Brito MJM, Alves M, Feldman LB. The implications of the accreditation process for patients from the perspective of nursing professionals. Enferm Glob 2012 jan;5:272-81.

14. Siman AG, Brito MJM, Carrasco MEL. Participation of the nurse manager in the hospital accreditation process. Rev Gaúcha Enferm 2014 jun;35(2):93-9.

15. Cunha FP, de Souza AA, Ferreira CO. Análise do endividamento de hospitais filantrópicos. XVII SemeAD - Seminários de Administração, 2014, São Paulo; Brazil.

16. Bonato VL. Quality management in health: improving customer care. Mundo Saúde 2011;35(5):319-31.

17. Rodrigues AVD, Vituri DW, Haddad MCL, Vannuchi MTO, de Oliveira WT. Responsiveness of the nursing service in the view of the client. Rev Esc Enferm USP 2012 dec; 46(6):1446-52.

18. Couto RHCT, Campos LI, Manzo BF, Brito MLM, Alves M. Study of nonconformities in nursing work: relevant evidence for hospital quality improvement. Aquichán 2014 Dec;14(4):582-593.

19. Siman AG, Cunha SGS, Martins ES, Brito MJM. Strategy of managerial work to achieve hospital accreditation. REME 2015 oct/dec;19(4): 815-822.

20. Santos JLG, et al. Practices of nurses in nursing care management and health: integrative review. Rev Bras Enferm 2013 mar/apr;66(2): 257-63.

21. Fernandes HMLG, Peniche ACG. Percepção da equipe de enfermagem do Centro Cirúrgico acerca da Acreditação Hospitalar em um Hospital Universitário. Rev Esc Enferm USP 2015 dec;49(spe):22-28.

CHAPTER 5

THE REGISTRATION OF HEALTH INFORMATION IN AN ACCREDITED HOSPITAL

Andréia Guerra Siman[1]
Simone Graziele Silva Cunha[2]
Marilane de Oliveira Fani
Amaro[3] Maria José Menezes
Brito[4]

INTRODUCTION

In the search for quality services, managers have made efforts to improve organizational processes with a view to market survival. To this end, they seek to improve their management policies, technologies and actions that drive the best development of their collaborators, focusing on customer satisfaction[1] .

From this perspective, to meet current demands, organizational managers have adopted Hospital Accreditation (HA), defined as an appropriate method to stimulate the integration and interrelation of the work process[2] .

The process of AH by the methodology of the National Accreditation Organization (ONA) is voluntary and carried out in institutions accredited by it, through diagnostic visits. The assessment of the hospital takes place *in loco*, generating a report, and the institution may be assessed as non-accredited or accredited; the latter being classified in three levels: Safety (level 1) called "Accredited"; Integrated Management (level 2) "Fully Accredited" and "Accredited with Excellence in Management (level 3)[3] . Through the evaluation, the non-conformities in the work are identified, as well as the harmony with the standards determined by the ONA.

It is pointed out that the assessment performed by the ONA allows the identification of inadequacies, increases the safety of the patient, professionals and managers of the organization, as well as provides recommendations for the work to occur in harmony, supported by teamwork and within the standards, offering greater reliability to the community[4] . In this sense, the AH process is directly linked to the managerial work at different levels, given that the various knowledge and actors need to articulate harmoniously to achieve the organization's objectives.

The principles of accreditation point to the need for the institution to use the Information System (IS) as a basis for generating data, indicators, rates and references, highlighting the need for data recording by professionals in order to generate information that will later be used for analysis, evaluation of activities and comparisons[5] . In this perspective, it is emphasized that there is a need to improve the records of assistance and management information in health, as a way to introduce advances in the work and to increase strategies for managers to develop their daily practices, in search of continuously improving the quality of assistance.

It is noteworthy that information is an essential element for the execution of the work of health professionals, because through its use it is possible to carry out the process of caring, managing and evaluating the actions[6] . Health information can be defined as a set of data that allows the visibility of certain problems or opportunities, when placed in a certain context and adequately provided .[7-8]

Thus, it is essential to improve health information records and have reliable information, since it enables the execution of an effective management of actions and, consequently, the achievement of excellence in quality, favors a better service, optimizes the chain of services and products, establishing a competitive differential[9] . Thus, records are instruments that contribute to the work of health professionals and can promote the continuity of care .[7-8]

In this context, professionals have been driven to seek improvement in the quality of information recorded intervening in the work. However, hospital institutions do not always have an information system, for structural, political or economic reasons. This fact contributes to the professional not having well structured, systematized and available information, frequently resulting in ineffective decision making. It is assumed that for information management it is necessary that all professionals feel responsible and involved and accountable for the production and use of the information record.

In view of the above, it is pointed out that through the implementation of the AH, it is possible that the work can develop effectively. It is a method that aims to change values and behaviors in the institution, valuing a better record of information, quality of care, safety, humanization and improvements in the service provided in the organizational environment, focusing on the search for excellence[10] .

Given the relevance of the need for health information records and the considerations presented, and also that this information subsidises the work and assists in meeting new organisational demands, the following question is posed: how does AH contribute to health information records?

Thus, this study aimed to analyze the contribution of accreditation in the recording of health information in a hospital accredited with "Excellence". This work is justified by the importance of the health record to perform a work with quality, structured and systematized, which meets the proposal of AH, to provide quality care with a view to meeting the demands of patients.

METHODS

This is a qualitative, descriptive research of the case study type. Qualitative research allows for an approximation of the individual's life reality, as well as to identify the society in which he/she is inserted[11] . The case study is one of the most adopted designs in qualitative research and aims to analyze a social unit, seeking to answer how and why the phenomena occur .[12]

The unit of analysis was a hospital, the context of the unique case in question, which is a large private hospital located in Belo Horizonte, MG, Brazil. This institution was successful in all stages of the accreditation process, and was appointed Excellence level by the National Accreditation Organization (ONA) in 2004. Thus, this hospital was chosen because it was the first hospital institution to be accredited at the Level of Excellence in Belo Horizonte. This hospital is a member of the National Association of Private Hospitals (ANAHP). It provides outpatient, inpatient and emergency care to the population, with spontaneous demand. It is open 24 hours a day, providing health insurance and private services. It has a total of 233 beds, distributed in two blocks: Block I, with 135 beds, and Block II, with 18 floors and 200 flats. Its characteristic is to be a science centre, electing as its main objective to develop medical assistance, teaching and research. To maintain the anonymity of the institution and facilitate the discussion and understanding of the results, the hospital was named "Hospital Gama".

Data collection was performed in 2011, through interviews with a semi-structured script, with managers who belonged to the intermediate management level. The inclusion criterion was that the subject should hold a management position and be inserted in hospital accreditation since its implementation, excluding those who did not experience the preparation for certification. Thus, 12 managers participated in the study, among them: five nurses, four physicians, two administrators and one accountant. The sample closure occurred through the use of information saturation. Saturation occurs when data become repetitive and redundant, so that they do not generate more information.[13]

The interviews took place at the subjects' workplace and were previously scheduled. The interviewees were informed about ethical and legal aspects. Upon authorization of the individuals, the interviews were recorded and transcribed in full, subsequently they were numbered according to the sequence in which they occurred, being identified with the letters GR (Manager).

The data collected were submitted to the Content Analysis[14], which comprised three phases: Pre-analysis: systematized organization of the material covering the floating reading; the constitution of the corpus, i.e., choice of documents taken into account to be submitted to analytical procedures; elaboration of categories, classes that gather a group of elements under a generic title, due to common characters and codification, which allows reaching the representation of the content. Exploration of the material: consisted of coding operations according to previously formulated rules, the categories having been confirmed. And finally, interpretation of content: it was intended to the treatment of results, occurring the condensation and highlighting of information for analysis in the light of the literature.

The study subjects signed the Informed Consent Form (ICF). It is noteworthy that all specifications of resolution 466/12 of the Ministry of Health were met. The research was approved by the Research Ethics Committee of the Hospital, scenario of this study, and by the Research Ethics Committee of UFMG, with opinion No. ETIC 0611.0.203.000-10.

Twelve managers participated in the study: five nurses, four physicians, two administrators and one accountant, with ages ranging from 29 to 58 years. The average time of work in the institution was 13.41 years, with maximum time of 19 years, and 91.66% of the managers have been in the institution for over 11 years. Regarding postgraduate studies, 100% of professionals took a postgraduate course: MBA Health Management, Hospital Administration, Executive MBA in Development, Human Resources Management, Intensive Care, Obstetrics Business Management, Finance Management, Logistics, Executive MBA, Hospital Administration, Auditing and People Management. Among the courses mentioned 10 (83.3%) are focused on the area of Management and Administration; and two (17.7%) refer to direct patient care.

The interpretative analysis of the interviews allowed the construction of the categories presented below.

Hospital accreditation and the recording of health information: changes in management work

Health information is established as a tool that guides managers in their work, allowing them to delimit the problem or opportunity, define actions and make inferences regarding the likelihood of the results. Thus, with the implementation of HA, the subjects claim that changes have occurred in the improvement of records and the way of dealing with information, as reported by GR2 and GR3.

We have to evaluate the viability of the businesses we have, with data, numerators, indicators, with a well-founded critical analysis. We have to have our actions more registered, for the accreditation programme. You have to register everything you do: what is good, what is bad, what you have done to improve. This is not a very common practice either. It was not a reality before. We still record less of what we do, but today we record better, in a more organised manner, with all our documentation of operational procedures. (GR2)

Accreditation brought the record of the actions taken. We planned, but did not record after implementation how it turned out [...] (GR3).

The care and administrative information started to be systematically recorded by the professionals after the implementation of AH, contributing for the developed managerial activities to be recorded and documented in a more organized way. The professionals experienced a change in the work process, since the accreditation enabled the performance of a previous analysis of the recorded information to plan and evaluate the actions.

The records have become more constant, but the interviewees recognise that this resource has not yet been used to its full potential, and that this activity needs to be improved.

It is noteworthy that with the registration of information, managers now have more grounds to carry out actions, promoting the planning of these actions through their analysis, thus reducing the degree of uncertainties.

Furthermore, accreditation is seen as a mobilizing point for the standardization of actions and consequently of work, as it introduces a standardization of documents and reports, according to the statements:

From 2004 (with the accreditation) we started to have several documents and to demand several work standardizations. If today we still have internal problems, we have to imagine what it would be like without this standardization. We know there is much room for improvement, but if today, even with the standardization defined, I have problems, what about before? (GR9)

What has changed is that since accreditation I have more instruments in a more standardised way. I know where to look for information and I know what I have. So, before, if they asked me for information, I had to search if I had this information, or sometimes create it, or sometimes it was informal, or I had to put together a report. Today, after accreditation, that availability you know the numbers more easily. You have the information more in real time and in a standard, registered form. (GR11)

The register provided organization of work and the exchange of information between sectors and among professionals, thus making available in time the necessary information for decision making. The subjects also perceived that the accreditation process, in addition to standardizing the work, organized the processes, providing ways to better measure the results and organizational performance, improving the quality of work and providing greater coverage and detailing of actions, making it possible to monitor them efficiently and effectively.

The SAME, the nickname was SOME. It was desperate. The computer part, how much the company developed! Today I have the electronic facility to relate to other sectors and speed up my work. The hospital made a very high investment in the IT area. Today we already have the entire SNA on the computer, the prescription. At the time of certification, we showed the whole system (GR1)

Today we have more tangible tools, which better direct the service [...] The processes were better described, generating a better quality of care and patient safety. (GR3)

Thus, the interviewees point out that there has been improvement in the IS and in health information records. However, despite mentioning that they use tools, they do not go into detail. They do not mention which information system they use to improve the speed and quality of information.

One thing that stands out is risk management, this was a gain. We started to record adverse events (GR10)

I see a lot of change regarding training records, formal evaluation, standardization, recording of non-compliance, indicators. Recording everything (GR8)

The managers of this study highlighted that, only with the AH, they started using management tools, such as: action plan; evaluation of indicators; customer-supplier chain; critical analysis of actions and risk matrix.

We have been improving the records. Presenting results through data, information. We realize that after we got involved with accreditation, we got involved with this (GR1)

When you work with indicators it is much better. Because you have a level, to really quantify what you are doing. Much better (GR12)

They emphasise the improvement in records for evaluation of results. Importantly, they begin to produce the information, disseminate it and make use of the information for decision making.

We work with indicators... and we pass everything on to our employees. We show the results and do an analysis and based on this analysis we propose improvement actions. Not only with the manager, but we tell our employees what the picture of our sector is within the company as a whole. (GR4)

This information is accessible to the professional, and not only to the manager, to assist them in the procedures and tasks performed, decision making, as well as to improve assistance, promoting improvement in the quality of work. It can be inferred that AH promotes a professional-social-ethical accountability of the collaborator who works in an accredited institution.

DISCUSSION

Due to the increasing production of data and information, health organizations have deployed an IS that can perform the exchange of information to facilitate the work, the realization of the health diagnosis, and promote the planning and evaluation of actions[15] .

In the hospital environment, in order to improve the quality of the services provided, the safety and efficiency of the processes, it is essential to invest in internal resources, among them in the IS, seeking to improve the availability of clinical information, workflows, complete information integration including supply, human resources, technical resources and billing, real-time management, collaborative care, connections with other care providers, as well as optimised planning[16] .

Moreover, it is pointed out that in health the IS is defined as an instrument that collects, processes, stores and distributes information that supports the decision-making process, with a view to promoting better management of actions in health services[6,17] .

Thus, through an effective IS it is possible to perform information management that contemplates the demands of the work in assistance and management, providing better care of patient demands and, consequently, the achievement of excellence in the quality of services[9] .

It is noteworthy that health information is considered a fundamental source for the planning and development of actions, generating the optimization of work, helping to improve the final result and improving patient care[9,18] . Besides, they seek to reflect the institutional reality, the health/disease process, administrative information, to know and quantify the problems, in order to establish efficient management models[15] . It is configured as a fundamental instrument in the work in health .[6]

In this sense, it is necessary to record this information in order to develop assistance focused on quality, promoting greater safety for professionals and the development of actions according to the demand presented by patients[19] . Which is intrinsically related to the principles of AH. The practice of recording information contributes to the safety of professionals, contributes to the continuity of care, decision making, creation of quality indicators, patient safety and provides greater coverage and detailing of actions .[8]

It is highlighted the creation of indicators in the organization. One of the components of an IS is the processing, which is formed by indicators. These are essential because they reflect on the institution's policy, organization, human resources, financial resources, health infrastructure, equipment and supplies. Besides, the health status, including information on mortality, morbidity, disability and well-being levels, being important for the services management and to guide the decision making[20] .

In addition, there are direct repercussions on the evaluation of results, as it organizes and facilitates the use of information, providing ways to measure the results and organizational performance, making a more accurate control of the actions performed. Therefore, improvements in records enrich the information and directly impact on service provision within the continuity of care.

In this context, it is emphasized that with the implementation of accreditation at Gama Hospital, there was an improvement in records, procedures and activities performed, as well as in the planning of care and management actions. It is noteworthy that the management of this information needs to be of an interdisciplinary nature, bringing together the different health professionals, because the individual and collective attitudes will be the key point for the transformation of different health care and management realities[21] .

Thus, AH can be highlighted as a trigger of changes in the work of health professionals, which reflects one of the objectives of the evaluation process cited in the ONA manual, which is to generate important information for its programming through the registration of events and activities[3] .

Action plan; evaluation of indicators; risk matrix, are instruments that have made it possible to improve performance, identify the weaknesses of the company and its strengths, maintaining the interoperability of information between sectors, processes and people[3] . This cultural change contributed so that the managerial activities were registered, thus promoting transformations in the way of dealing with information in the institution.

It is identified a recognition of managers regarding the importance of recording health information, not identifying this task as bureaucratic or that increases the workload, but above all, as a facilitator of the development of a more organized work, with more tangible data, reflecting on the quality of care. However, there must be not only the recognition of the importance of the record as to perform it constantly, requiring the participation and involvement of all employees of the institution. It is essential that professionals have complete, updated and reliable information to perform their function in a planned manner .[17]

It should be noted that according to WHO, some actions should be taken to improve information, such as local quality control and verification of the use of information, the use of clear definitions for information elements, and especially refresher training and frequent feedback to those who collect and use the data[20] .

It is pointed out that the AH contributed to the managers seeking to organize the services and standardize the actions, generating a performance with more security and autonomy in the decision-making process. Thus, it was possible to identify changes in the daily work of managers, since there was a standardization of processes through the systematization of the information record. This fact led to an improvement in communication between managers and sectors, teamwork and constant evaluation and review of processes. The information became available on time, promoting a planned and quality work.

It can be inferred that with hospital accreditation the managers started to plan their actions better and to work in an articulated manner with the others, losing the character of fragmented actions and without reflection on the daily routine.

Accreditation favored the registration of information at Gama Hospital, and subsidized decision-making in health, with a focus on continuous improvement. It is worth highlighting that the accreditation process is characterized as a continuous, periodic and stimulating process[3] , allowing the achievement of new quality levels for organizational performance, and should be encouraged and developed in the largest number of institutions, with a view to enabling quality care for the entire population.

A limitation of the study was to have carried out data collection seven years after the first certification, which required participants to recall old facts. In addition, it was carried out in a single institution, and, therefore, its results cannot be generalized.

CONCLUSIONS

The registration of information allows professionals to have a better visibility of their current and future challenges and opportunities, contributing to the performance of a work consistent with the respective reality of the institution. Pelo estudo foi possível identificar que o processo de AH proporcionou avanços importantes nesta construção, contribuindo com a organização dos registros em saúde e entraizar uma cultura de valorização do registro da informação em um hospital acreditado com "Excelência".

It was possible to identify that the AH brought new configurations to the work of the professionals inserted in the organization, bringing benefits to the institution and its social actors, with repercussions in the information record, reflecting on the management practice carried out.

It is noticed that hospital managers involved in the accreditation program have sought an improvement in hospital information records, which significantly contributes to a planned and discussed decision-making, that is, it increased the probability of the decision-making process being assertive. Thus, this study contributed to collaborate with the analysis of the accreditation process, showing that it provides improvements in the health record, contributes to the organization of nursing work and its links with assistance to achieve less stressful and quality paths.

The objective of the study was achieved and the methodology was adequate. Further studies focused on the analysis of the quality of information are suggested. Therefore, further discussions on accreditation and its contributions throughout the health system, linking the Health Information System and technological changes in hospitals are essential.

REFERENCES

1. Duarte MSM, Silvino ZR. Acreditação Hospitalar x Qualidade dos serviços de saúde. Rev. Pesq. cuid. fundam. online. [internet]. 2010 [accessed on: 2014 Nov 26]; 2(Ed.suppl.):182-185. Available from: file:///C:/Users/bolsistas_2/Downloads/858-6364-1-PB.pdf

2. Maziero VG, Spiri WC. Significance of the hospital accreditation process for nurses of a state public hospital. Rev. Eletr. Enf. [internet]. 2013 [accessed 2014 Dec 02];15(1):121-129. Available at: http://dx.doi.org/10.5216/ree.v15i1.14757

3. National Accreditation Organization. Manual de Organizações Prestadoras de Serviços Hospitalares. Brasília: ONA; 2010.

4. Siman AG, Brito MJM, Carrasco MEL. Participation of the nurse manager in the hospital accreditation process. Rev. Gaúcha Enferm. [internet]. 2014 [accessed on: 2014 Dec 02];35(2):93-99. Disponível em: http://www.scielo.br/pdf/rgenf/v35n2/pt_1983-1447-rgenf-35-02-00093.pdf

5. Ministério da Saúde (BR). Secretaria de Assistência à Saúde. Acreditação Hospitalar. Manual Brasileiro de Acreditação Hospitalar. Secretaria de Assistência à Saúde. 3ª ed. rev. e atual. Brasília: Ministério da Saúde; 2002.

6. Marin HF. Health information systems: general considerations. J.Health Inform. [Internet]. 2010 [accessed: 2014 Dec 14];2(1):20-24. Available from: http://www.jhi-sbis.saude.ws/ojs-jhi/index.php/jhi-sbis/article/viewFile/4/52

7. Almeida MCV, Cezar-Vaz MR, Figueiredo PP, Cardoso LS, Sant'Anna CF, Bonow CA. Registro em saúde como instrumento no processo de trabalho das equipes de saúde da família. Cienc. Cuid. Saude. [Internet]. 2009 [accessed 2014 Dec 14]; 8(3):305-312. Available at: http://www.periodicos.uem.br/ojs/index.php/CiencCuidSaude/article/viewFile/9009/4994

8. Sousa PAF, Sasso GTMD, Barra DCC. Contributions of electronic records for patient safety in intensive care: an integrative review. Texto Contexto Enferm. [Internet]. 2012 [accessed on: 2014 Dec 14];21(4):971-979. Available at:

http://www.scielo.br/pdf/tce/v21n4/en_30.pdf

9. Pereira SR, Paiva PB, Souza PRS, Siqueira G, Pereira AR. Sistema de Informação para Gestão Hospitalar. J.Health Inform. [Internet]. 2012 [accessed on: 2014 Dec 14];4(4):170-175. Available from: file:///C:/Users/bolsistas_2/Downloads/206-1096-1-PB.pdf

10. Manzo BF, Ribeiro HCTC, Brito MJM, Alves M. As percepções dos profissionais de saúde sobre o processo de acreditação hospitalar. Rev. enferm. UERJ. [Internet]. 2011 [accessed on: 2014 Dec 14];19(4):571-576. Available at: http://www.facenf.uerj.br/v19n4/v19n4a11.pdf

11. Minayo MCS. The challenge of knowledge: qualitative health research. 13a ed. São Paulo: Hucitec; 2013.

12. Yin RK. Case study: planning and methods. 4a ed. Porto Alegre: Bookman; 2010.

13. Polit DF, Beck CT. Fundamentals of nursing research: evaluating evidence for nursing practice. Trad. de Denise Regina de Sales. 7a ed. Porto Alegre: Artmed; 2011.

14. Bardin L. Análise de conteúdo. 5a ed. Lisboa: Edições 70; 2011.

15. Carreno I, Moreschi C, Marina B, Hendges DJB, Rempel C, Oliveira MMC. Analysis of the use of information from the Basic Care Information System (SIAB): an integrative review. Ciênc. saúde coletiva [Internet]. 2015 [accessed on: 2015 May 15]; 20(3):947-956 Available from: http://www.scielo.br/pdf/csc/v20n3/1413-8123-csc-20-03-00947.pdf

16. Lovis C, Ball M, Boyer C, Elkin PL, Ishikawa K, Jaffe C, et al. Hospital and Health Information Systems - Current Perspectives. Contribution of the IMIA Health Information Systems Working Group. Yearb Med Inform. [Internet]. 2011 [accessed: 2014 Dec 14];6(1):73-82. Available from: file:///C:/Users/bolsistas_2/Downloads/unige_21583_attachment01.pdf

17. Pinochet LHC. Trends in Information Technology in Health Management. The Health World. [Internet]. 2011 [accessed 2014 Dec 14]; 35(4):382-394. Available at: http://saocamilo-sp.br/pdf/mundo_saude/88/03_TendenciasdeTecnologia.pdf

18. Barbosa DCM, Forster AC. Sistemas de informação em saúde: a perspectiva e a avaliação dos profissionais envolvidos na atenção primária à saúde de Ribeirão Preto. Cad de Saúde Coletiva. [Internet]. 2010 [accessed 2014 Dec 14]; 18(3):424-433. Available at: http://www.researchgate.net/profile/Debora_Cristina_Barbosa/publication/275346752_Sistemas_de_Informao_em_Sade_a_perspectiva_e_a_avaliao_dos_profissionais_envolvidos_na_Ateno_Primária_Sade_de_Ribeiro_Preto_So_Paulo/links/5539bbf30cf247b858814774.pdf

19. Lucena AF. Nursing process: interfaces with the hospital accreditation process. Rev. Gaúcha Enferm. [Internet]. 2013 [accessed on: 2014 Dec 15];34(4):8-9. Available from: file:///C:/Users/bolsistas_2/Downloads/45306-183384-1-PB.pdf

20. World Health Organization. Framework and standards for country health information systems. 2nd ed. Geneva; 2008.

21. Moraes IHS, Gómez MNG. Information and health informatics: contemporary kaleidoscope of health. Ciênc. Saúde Coletiva. [Internet]. 2007 [accessed 2014 Dec 14];12(3):553-565. Available at: http://www.scielo.br/pdf/csc/v12n3/02.pdf

CHAPTER 6

HOSPITAL ACCREDITATION: THE PROCESS FROM THE MANAGERS' PERSPECTIVE

Andreia Guerra Siman, Maria José Menezes Brito, Marilane de Oliveira Fani Amaro, Amanda Aparecida Correa Martins Machado

SUMMARY:

Objective: to understand the perception of managers of a hospital about hospital accreditation. **Método:** estudo de caso qualitativo realizado em um hospital acreditado em Excelência. Os dados foram coletados por meio de entrevistas semiestruturada com 12 gerentes de diferentes categorias e realizada a análise de conteúdo. **Resultados: os gerentes** percebem o processo de acreditação como de fundamental importância para a instituição, profissionais e pacientes. Reconhecem como positivas as mudanças nas estruturas, nos processos e nos resultados para uma assistência de qualidade, desde que todos os colaboradores se envolvam nesse processo. **Considerações finais: As mudanças** físicas, estruturais, de processos e de melhorias na instituição são como reestruturação para oferecer uma assistência de melhor qualidade. It was also possible to identify the strong educational approach of accreditation, perceiving the accreditation process as a generator of professional knowledge and strategy to achieve quality.

Keywords: Quality management; Quality of health care; Accreditation; Hospitals.

INTRODUCTION

The focus on the value of the service provided of good quality, prioritizing innovation, knowledge and execution of the strategy, achieves shareholder returns superior to those of companies with eyes only on the investor. Management in the health area seeks solutions to growing challenges: to associate quality of care with the reduction or at least control of increasingly higher costs, not necessarily associated with excellence

Organizations in all sectors of the economy, including health, are adopting management models focused on quality to succeed in the face of new demands imposed by the competitive market and by the internal organizational environment. Management in the health area seeks solutions for growing challenges: to associate quality of care with the reduction or at least control of increasingly higher costs, not necessarily associated with excellence.[1] The quality of a service can be defined as a set of characteristics to satisfy explicit or implicit needs of customers and the organisation.[2]

In this sense, the World Health Organisation (WHO) recommends the adoption of the Brazilian Accreditation Programme, which classifies institutions into quality levels, promoting learning based on the value given to a reality in the light of a reference or standard, followed by a systematic assessment.[3,4] This programme has been carried out in Brazil since 1999 by the National Accreditation Organisation (ONA), which is a non-governmental organisation that aims to implement a permanent process of assessment and certification of the quality of health institutions, encouraging the continuous improvement of the quality of care, on a national scale.[5]

For this purpose, levels are established to demonstrate the qualification level of the organization: level 1 refers to the basic quality requirements; level 2 refers to the evidences of planning in the organization and level 3, contemplates the continuous improvement policies in the hospital structures[6] . This classification is performed by a team of evaluators of the Accreditation Institutions Accredited by ONA, which are based on pre-established standards in the ONA Manual of Health Service Providers, seeking to identify *on site* evidence of quality in the institutions under evaluation process.[5]

Accreditation is evaluated by many authors as an important process in the quality of health care and continuous improvement of services.[7;8;9] In a recent study it was concluded that quality management in ONA requirements contributed to increase financial efficiency and effectiveness, organize processes, meet customer requirements, develop and satisfy employees, leading to improved results and hospital quality.[8] However, the impact of standards-based external evaluation models varies according to their purpose, standards, procedures and incentives. In this sense, another study "Methods for evaluating the response to quality improvement strategies" signaled that private hospitals with higher levels of safety were associated more with accreditation than with ISO certification, but that both systems were significantly better than nothing.[10]

In this perspective, the achievement of accreditation demands great effort from hospital managers, who aim at developing knowledge, competences and abilities in the institution's collaborators that provide continuous improvement cycles of hospital quality. The great differential of the organizations is in the scope of the quality and performance of their collaborators, the technology and the structure of the organizations may have little meaning if the people do not feel committed with the quality, especially in what refers to the fulfillment of the customers' needs.[11] Thus, managers should bear in mind that employees are the core of the quality policy, having an essential role in ensuring and maintaining the process.[3]

Thus, this study aimed to understand the accreditation process from the perspective of hospital managers. From the results achieved, it is expected to collaborate with the reflections on the accreditation process and help professionals, especially managers, to face the challenges of the accreditation process, thus ensuring the provision of quality service.

METHOD

This is a case study of qualitative nature, which applies to the study of history, relationships, representations, beliefs, perceptions and opinions, products of the interpretations that social subjects make about how they live, build their artifacts, feel and think.[12] The case study aims to investigate contemporary phenomena in their real context, being characterized by deep and exhaustive study of one or a few objects, to allow broad and detailed knowledge of it.[13]

The study was conducted in a large private hospital in the capital of Minas Gerais, Belo Horizonte, Brazil. This hospital was accredited with the level of excellence, achieving success in all stages of the Accreditation process in 2006. The choice of research participants was intentionally made, excluding professionals who were not part of the institution and the Accreditation process since its implementation.

Data collection was carried out through interviews, scheduled personally with the participants, from April to May 2011, with a semi-structured script, with 12 managers of different professional categories and hierarchical levels. Nurses, physicians and administrators participated in the interviews. The criterion of information saturation was used to delimit the interviews, which advocates the suspension of the inclusion of new participants when the data obtained begin to present, in the researcher's assessment, a certain redundancy or repetition, considered not relevant to persist in data collection.[14]

The questions assessed aspects such as managerial activities, managerial actions in the AH Process, as well as the manager's role in this process and facilitating and hindering aspects. The interviews lasted an average of 30 minutes, were audio-recorded with the subjects' prior consent, transcribed in full, and numbered according to the sequence in which they occurred and with the acronym GR (Manager). The data collected were subjected to content analysis seeking to achieve a deeper interpretation of the phenomenon, in addition to exceeding the merely descriptive scope of the manifest content of the message.[15]

The data analysis was performed, around three chronological poles: pre-analysis, exploration of the material and treatment of the results with thematic analysis, which represents a set of techniques for analysis of communications that aim to obtain knowledge relating to these messages.[15] The thematic analysis works on the beam of a given subject, and was performed in three phases, being the first: pre-analysis, also known as "floating reading", was given by the organization of what was going to be analyzed. Second: exploration of the material, the material was coded, a cut of the text was made and then we classified and aggregated the data, organizing them into theoretical categories. And third, treatment of results, where the raw data was worked, allowing highlighting the information obtained, which will be interpreted in the light of the literature.[15]

Regarding ethical aspects, the study was submitted and approved by the Ethics and Research Committee of the institution where this study was carried out and by the Research Ethics Committee of UFMG, with Opinion No. ETIC 0611.0.203.000-10. All professionals participating in the study signed the Informed Consent Form.

RESULTS AND DISCUSSION

Hospital Accreditation: a path with no turning back

From the managers' perspective, accreditation systematises work processes and makes it possible to monitor institutional results. What was exposed can be verified in the following speech:

> *When the accreditation came, we had the opportunity to systematise the work, the opportunity to better monitor the results. So, accreditation is very good, its maintenance is hard work, but when you are accredited it is a path with no return. You can't work any other way, without follow-up. We go through the difficulties of implementation, but after that we just have to reap the results* (GR6)

Quality is a philosophy of life before being a philosophy of action,[11] expression that ratifies the aforementioned statement, that the quality policy when adopted by the institution is a path with no return. When experiencing the results that the standard adopted by the accreditation provides to the institution and to the patients, the organization does not accept being inserted in another perspective other than the quality perspective. The process must be continuous, so that it is not enough to do it sporadically, the quality standard must always be kept active. From the managers' perspective, hospital accreditation can be analyzed as a positive experience, demonstrating that it is a strategy for the institution to remain in the competitive market, as a way to survive and also as a way to stand out from other hospital institutions.

> *Accreditation is an extremely valid process. Today the patient looks for an accredited hospital. The media publicises it, knowledge has increased and people already know what accreditation is* (GR3)

This idea reinforces the view that the process of Hospital Accreditation favours the trust of the community, a stimulating factor for its growth and acceptance.[6]

The hospital accreditation is based on three pillars of quality: structure, process and result.[16] The hospital institution, as a health service provider, when entering the process of Hospital Accreditation, undergoes important modifications and restructuring to offer better quality care. Through this study, it was possible to understand, from the perspective of managers of various categories, the changes generated inside the hospital in terms of structure.

> *We really started to change some actions towards certification, the biggest adjustment was in the physical, structural part of the hospital ... the hospital has been built for a long time, we had to adapt a lot of things, and there are still many things that we are going to adapt, we certified with the planning already in the implementation phase.* (GR1)

Regarding the structure, the institution must meet the requirements that contemplate the basic requirements of quality in customer care, with human resources compatible with the complexity, adequate qualification (habilitation) of the professionals and responsible technicians with corresponding qualification for the areas of operation. Besides, it needs to offer safe care to customers and for this to occur, it is essential to control risks to patients.[4] In this context, the risk in health services is attributable to the structure, work processes, products and health technologies[17] and the error is related to two types of failures, which are one of execution, when the action is not done correctly as intended and the other of planning, in which the planned action is not correct.[18] Thus, health care, which is by principle a risk activity, presents the need to achieve safety management in the hospital environment, in order to improve and increase the quality of its services.

Managers also reported changes in work processes, as presented in the statements below:

> *We started to work in a more synchronized way, nobody imposes anything anymore, it is discussed and agreed. Each sector sets up the client-supplier chain and we discuss how we want to receive the product and how we want to supply the product, so it is agreed. (GR10)*

> *In addition to the accreditation bringing us security in our work and also brought the necessary documentation. Today all our documents are registered in a matrix, all our activities are documented. The records are periodically reviewed, the operational procedures, and we also work with indicators to monitor the performance of our work, in addition to periodic critical analysis and internal and external audits that make us maintain our work properly. (GR6)*

In this focus, the processes related to the organisation are care activities performed for a patient, actions often linked to an outcome, as well as activities related to the infrastructure. That is, they are operational techniques, which are essentially concerned with the performance of the health professionals' work, from a technical point of view, in the conduction of care, diagnosis, therapy and their interaction with patients through the preparation of clinical records, diagnosis, treatment, evolution and transfer of clients.[19]

It is noteworthy that the accreditation process brought changes in the actions of managers. The developed activities started to be registered and documented with more organisation and in a systematic way, using management tools such as the risk matrix. These are demands of the process that offer professional security. In addition, the institution needs to establish the indicators that will measure the work process in a systematic way, to be used later as a form of evaluation of the services offered.

The indicators measure quantitative aspects that can be used as a tool to monitor and evaluate the quality of care provided to the patient and the activities of support services. Thus, the monitoring and evaluation of these indicators are essential for the development of continuing education and training programs, thus favoring the improvement of the care provided.[19]

In relation to continuous improvement cycles, corresponding to level three of management excellence, participants reported:

The statement emphasizes the importance of continuity in the process even after the institution receives the accreditation certificate. It is the management identifying opportunities for advancement, giving continuity to the process thinking about improvements and results. These strategic objectives contemplate perspectives that contribute to the achievement of the organisation's vision of the future.

Accreditation Process: professional knowledge focused on organisational results

Hospital quality depends primarily on the action of its professionals, through the knowledge acquired in the academy and throughout their professional life. Thus, the institutions are increasingly investing in human development, aiming at adding value both for the professionals and for the organisation, characterising the conciliation of organisational and professional interests. In the hospital accreditation process, the investment in human development is fundamental. Moreover, the participation of all professionals is essential for the success of the "quality management", because the high performance of the institution depends on the commitment and collaboration of those involved in the process.[20]

In this sense, managers are responsible for leading and conducting the employees under their responsibility for continuous improvement in the accreditation process. However, it seems that they are not prepared for such a function, as demonstrated in the statements below, in which the research participants report that accreditation generates personal knowledge to deal with professional issues of everyday work.

The hospital accreditation process aims to improve the quality of care. Quality is everything that adds value to work or relationships and is directly linked to the productivity of the institution, involving human relationships and professional and personal development.[21]

In this context, it is worth highlighting the importance of the professional training of those who will experience the Accreditation process. Through a training imbued with the principles of quality, it is possible to develop professional competences related mainly to motivation and leadership, important tools to achieve quality work.[7] In this way, the competences acquired by health professionals are essential for the feasibility of Accreditation; knowledge, leadership, vulnerability and experiences acquired in the day-to-day organizational practices. [7] The idea is expressed in the reports:

> *And I took the company from the beginning of its whole organization, awareness... I think it grew a lot, not only structurally, but intellectually. Things become easier and working with results is a revolution within the company, right, because it is a revolution, but now I see results* (GR4)

> *I think that the accreditation process improves because it brings you knowledge and shows you the sum, because you have to try to improve your day to day work.* (GR7)

> *Accreditation came to audit what we already work, but it adds a lot because they are experiences from other institutions, experiences of innovations, which add value to what you already do and here in the laboratory we were fortunate to have auditors from our area. So it is a very big growth, we receive suggestions for improvement and it ends up being a two-way street, we receive important information from them and pass on to them the way we understood that manual.* (GR6)

Thus, it is possible to state that the generation of professional knowledge is the way to achieve the organisational results to reach accreditation. Because, unlike traditional assessment processes, it has a strong educational approach, based on the reflection of the professional practice, which leads to the elaboration of standards of excellence in performance. As it is a mainly reflective process, it always reveals new ways of visualising and acting on the institution's problems.[22]

Hospital Accreditation: guarantee of quality?

Health care is complex and hospital accreditation aims at quality improvement. The hospital accreditation is not the goal, the goal respects to the achievement of the quality improvement of the several sectors that integrate the hospital. The hospital accreditation must be considered as a method which develops evaluation instruments for the continuous improvement of the quality of the care for patients and the organisational performance, offering the community's trust in their hospital.[4]

However, does hospital accreditation guarantee the quality of care? It is relevant to reflect that the hospital accreditation process is a management strategy, where the organization that adheres to the process commits to quality and has the possibility, not the guarantee, of providing quality care. The certification by itself does not guarantee the quality of the services rendered, it only indicates that the services are able to produce it.[13] For this, it is necessary to create a favourable culture in order to materialise this commitment.

From this perspective, hospital accreditation is a strategy to achieve quality. In this study, the meaning of hospital accreditation as continuous improvement emerged from the statements, which indicates the commitment with quality and not only with hospital accreditation:

With the accreditation issue, our goal is quality. We did not want to work for accreditation, we wanted to work with quality every day, it is not a matter of doing everything nicely and leaving everything organized because today there is an audit, no, it is to get everyone into the culture, into the day-to-day that we have to have quality. (GR10)

Accreditation is not about getting a certificate, it is an organisational maturing, I think that the companies that have not sought this are losing a lot of time, time for survival in the market, because to achieve this we have to bring people to know, understand not the method, the methodology, the manuals, but understand that this will be good for the institution in general, reduce rework, reduce waste, costs, optimise processes, resources that we have to do more and more with less. (GR7)

What we understand of the process is that if you incorporate a quality management program as a day-to-day routine, as it is part of your day-to-day. You don't have to build it a month before or two months before, and we have already reached this level, of incorporating it into the routine of quality on a daily basis. (GR2) Analysing the statements, the managers' relations with quality and

continuous improvement, which goes beyond an accreditation certificate. The interviewees express that the central focus is quality, which is in line with the literature, in the sense of fixing quality in the day-to-day work. Furthermore, they are understanding the importance of joining the accreditation process. The professional maturity and assimilation of the process reflects in doing it once only, avoiding rework, wear and tear and cost. The health services present high costs characterized by the bad quality, high expenses with morbidity, besides inefficient processes and rework.[23] It is in the perspective of reverting this situation that hospital Accreditation has a real meaning.

It is noteworthy that besides the accreditation process avoiding rework, it is a periodic process, i.e., it is not an acquired state, there are steps to be taken and it must be a periodic process to avoid quality being considered an acquired state instead of being a permanent process.[13] What is exposed in the following speech:

I think that the process has been maturing more and more, and making people, managers and the user itself more aware of the importance of doing the right thing the first time, focusing on the safety of the environment, focusing on the safety of people, on safety in a hospital, on safety of care above all. (GR7)

The accreditation process is great, but it demands much more work from nurses, so today there are more stages, so is the accreditation, it increases the quality of service, but it also increases the volume of services, it certainly does. (GR3)

This process may result in the maturation and involvement of people, the necessary commitment to achieve quality. However, when expressing the accreditation process as a periodic process it was also observed that some managers explain the demand for work, the increase in the volume of services, not only of managers, but of the entire team.

> *It generated a lot of demand from the service, both from management, coordination and supervision, and from nursing technicians and assistants as well, because they had to organize more, bureaucratize things more, like the SAE. The SAE is great, but it demands much more work from nurses* (GR4)

Similarly in a study carried out,[3] the professionals reported as difficulty factors, the lack of time, work overload and charging. The time is considered short because the bureaucratic part of Accreditation consumes a large part of the professionals' working day; the work overload comes from the need to pay attention to the bureaucracy, in addition to common tasks, while the charge falls on the urgency for quality and perfection. Thus, the overload demanded by the increase in productivity may weaken the professionals, to the extent that they do not have the opportunity to build and conquer human development.[9]

Still in relation to implementing the accreditation process and improvement actions, some managers positively express the adjustments focused on the patient. Thus, during the journey to achieve accreditation, hospital organizations ensure, based on certain standards, the quality of services provided and this includes improvements in the institution:

> *They look at what you are offering the patient, the external area, accommodation, identify the validity of everything, it's something that nobody pays for, it's quality, safety for the patient, for the hospital and for the professional.* (GR3)

> *With the accreditation we really started to change some actions towards certification, the SAME - the nickname of the SAME - was Some, because you used to go in and it was hopeless, today you go in and find the paper as if you had just come down, you find all the papers, and we can see how far the company has come.* (GR1)

The statement reflects the hospital's preparation for accreditation. In this sense, it emerges that in the accreditation process the preparation of the hospital is very important, where all work processes are reviewed and improvement actions are implemented. Thus, quality improvements are a set of actions whose focus is the patient. The concept of quality is based on the balance between structure, process and result of a system, which certifies that the level of quality is also influenced by the structure that the organisation offers.[16] In this sense, the approach to quality assurance should consider the need and expectation of patients. Thus, hospital accreditation may not guarantee the quality of the care provided, but offers resources to achieve this quality and a quantitative perspective in health programs and services, which is fundamental for the planning, organization, direction, evaluation and control of the activities developed.[19] **FINAL CONSIDERATIONS**

Hospitals seek new care and management models to achieve results with fewer resources and with care focused on the patient's needs, besides the quality of services offered with safety for the patient and the professional. This study sought to deepen the reflection on the process of hospital accreditation from the perspective of managers, and it was possible to identify that hospital managers perceive the accreditation process in a positive and valid way, as a process that brings changes in the developed activities, in the behavior and in the commitment to quality.

In this sense, the results showed that the manager perceives the accreditation process as a perspective of continuity, of importance not only for the institution but also for patients and professionals involved. The managers perceive positively the physical and structural changes, of processes and improvements in the institution; as restructuring to offer better quality care. From the managers' point of view, it was also possible to identify the strong educational approach of accreditation, perceiving the accreditation process as a generator of professional knowledge and also as a strategy to achieve quality, but without the commitment of the actors involved, there is no guarantee of quality care.

The hospital accreditation showed to be a methodology of changes and transformations in an organization that go beyond structural changes. The Accreditation process has repercussions of educational transformations, with knowledge in indicators, technologies, work processes providing managers with the acquisition of new skills and new competences in a dynamic way.

To conclude, the methodology adopted was adequate, the proposed objectives were achieved, collaborating with the reflections on the Accreditation process in hospital institutions, in light of the managers' perceptions. However, it is evident the need for further studies on hospital accreditation aiming to raise the necessary changes to offer a more humanized and excellence of care.

REFERENCES

1- Fernandes HS, Silva E, Neto AC, Pimenta LA, Knobel E. Gestão em terapia intensiva: Conceitos e inovações. Rev. Bras. Clin. Med. 2011; 9(2):129-37.

2- - Lobo RN. Gestão da Qualidade. São Paulo (SP): Érica; 2010.

3- Manzo BF, Ribeiro HCTC, Brito MJM, Alves M. As percepções dos profissionais de saúde sobre o processo de acreditação hospitalar. Rev. Enferm. UERJ. 2011; 19(4):571-6.

4- Novaes HM. The process of accreditation of health services. Rev Adm Saúde. 2007; 9(37):133-40.

5-National Accreditation Organization (ONA). Get to know ONA. 2011. Available at: https://www.ona.org.br/Pagina/20/Conheca-a-ONA. Accessed 10 Jun 2017.

6- Lima SBS, Erdmann AL. A enfermagem no processo da acreditação hospitalar em um serviço de urgência e emergência. Acta Paul Enferm. 2006; 19(3):271-8.

7- Siman AG, Brito MJM, Carrasco MEL. Participação do enfermeiro gerente no processo de acreditação hospitalar. Rev Gaúcha Enferm. 2014; 35(2): 93-9.

8- Labbadia LL, Matsushita MS, Piveta VM, Viana TA, Cruz FSL. O processo de Acreditação Hospitalar e a participação da enfermeira. Rev enferm UERJ. 2004; 12(1): 83-7.

9- Porto IS, Rego MMS. Implantation of quality systems in hospital institutions: implications for nursing. ACTA Paul Enfermagem. 2005;18 (4):434-8.

10- Shaw C, Bruneau C, Kutryba B, Guido J, Sunol R. Towards hospital standardization in Europe. International Journal for Quality in Health Care [Internet] 2010 Aug [accessed 2017 Jul 1]; 22(4):244-9. Available at: http://intqhc.oxfordjournals.org.

11- Mezomo JC. Gestão da qualidade na saúde: princípios básicos. 1. ed. São Paulo: Loyola, 2001. 301 p.

12- Minayo MCS. The Challenge of Knowledge: Qualitative Research in Health. 11ª ed. São Paulo (SP): Hucitec; 2010.

13- Yin RK. Case studies: planning and methods. Translation by Daniel Grassi. 5a ed. Porto Alegre (RS): Brookman; 2015.

14-Fontanella BJM, Ricas J, Turato ER. Saturation sampling in qualitative health research: theoretical contributions. Cad Saúde Pública. 2008; 24(1): 17-27.

15- Bardin L. Content analysis. Translation by Luis Antero Reto and Augusto Pinheiro. São Paulo: Edições 70/Livraria Martins Fontes; 1979.

16- Donabedian, Avedis. Evaluating the Quality of Medical Care. 1969. The Milbank quarterly 83.4 (2005):691-729. Available at: www.periodicos.capes.gov.br. Accessed: 22 May 2017.

17- Anvisa. Agência Nacional de Vigilância Sanitária. 2° Relatório sobre o Sistema Brasileiro de Acreditação. Brasília: ANVISA, 2006.

18- Schwappach DLB, Engaging patients as vigilant partners in safety: A systematic review. Medical care research and review. 2010; 67(2): 119-148.

19- Bittar OJNV. Indicadores de qualidade e quantidade em saúde. Rev Adm Saúde. 2001;12 (4):21-8.

20- Puccini PT; Cecilio LCO. The humanization of services and the right to health. Caderno de Saúde Pública. 2004;20(5): 1342-53.

21- Bonato VL. Gestão em saúde: programas de qualidade em hospitais. 1. ed. São Paulo: Icone, 2007. 119 p.

22- Rooney AL; Ostenber PR. Licensure, Accreditation and certification: approaches to health services quality. Quality assurance project, Center for Human Services - CHS. USA: USAID, 1999. 64 p.

23- Camillo NRS, Oliveira JLC, Bellucci Jr JA, Cervilheri AH, Haddad MCFL, Matsuda LM. Accreditation in a public hospital: perceptions of a multidisciplinary team. Rev Bras Enferm [Internet]. 2016;69(3):423-30. DOI: http://dx.doi.org/10.1590/0034-7167.2016690306i

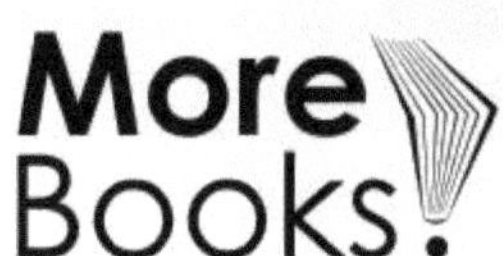

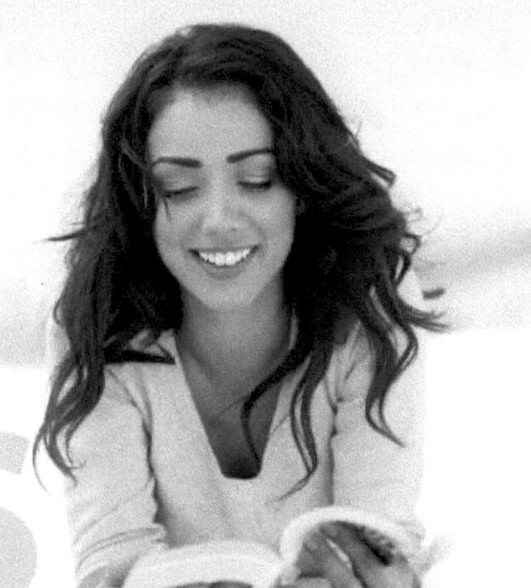

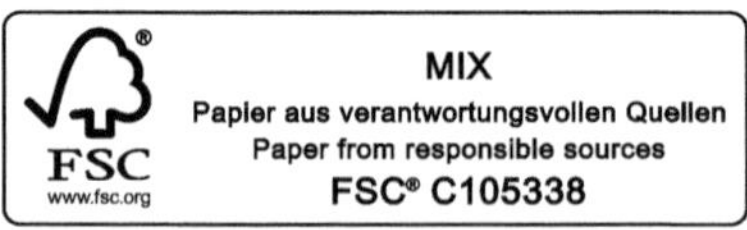

Printed by Books on Demand GmbH, Norderstedt / Germany